EMPOWERING THE CHILD WITH CEREBRAL PALSY

A GUIDE FOR PARENTS AND FAMILIES

Dr. A. MITRA, MBBS, MD, DMI.

Disclaimer:

The information provided in this book, "Empowering the Child with Cerebral Palsy," is intended for educational purposes only. While every effort has been made to ensure accuracy and relevance, readers are advised to consult healthcare professionals for personalized advice and treatment options tailored to individual circumstances. The author and publisher disclaim any liability arising directly or indirectly from the use or application of the contents of this book.

DEDICATION

This is a tribute to the heroes in parents and families who, with their ceaseless love, resilience, and commitment, provide children with cerebral palsy the strength to overcome obstacles and flourish. The steadfast bravery and perseverance of these families serve as an inspiration to us all.

CONTENTS

- Transitioning to Adult Healthcare Systems
- Patient Autonomy and Shared Decision-Making
- Importance of Regular Medical Checkups
- Early Detection of Potential Health Concerns
- Sexuality and Relationship Education
- Promoting Healthy Body Image and Self-Esteem
- Addressing Individual Needs

- Understanding Government Programs & Benefits
- Health Insurance Considerations & Advocacy
- Educational Funding & Scholarships
- Planning for Long-Term Care Needs
- Estate Planning & Financial Security

- Coping with Stress and Managing Difficult Emotions
- Importance of Self-Care for Parents & Siblings
- Finding Support Groups & Respite Care Options
- Maintaining Strong Family Relationships
- Celebrating Achievements and Milestones

- The Unique Role of Siblings
- Acknowledging and Addressing Difficult Emotions
- Communication and Open Dialogue
- Supporting Sibling Development

- Identifying Your Child's Passions and Interests
- Promoting Independence and Self-Advocacy
- Fostering a Positive Future Outlook

ACKNOWLEDGMENTS

I extend heartfelt gratitude to all who contributed to "Empowering the Child with Cerebral Palsy." Thanks to the courageous children and families for sharing their experiences. Deep appreciation to healthcare professionals, therapists, educators, and researchers for their dedication. Special thanks to colleagues, friends, and mentors for their unwavering support and feedback. Gratitude also to the publishing team for their hard work. This book is a testament to a compassionate community dedicated to empowering children with cerebral palsy and fostering inclusivity.

Thank you all.

Dr. A. Mitra

1. UNDERSTANDING CEREBRAL PALSY

Cerebral Palsy (CP) in simple words

Imagine the brain as the boss of the body, directing the muscles' actions. In cerebral palsy, there is a glitch in how the brain's messages are sent. This glitch can occur before birth, during birth, or shortly after. Due to these mixed-up messages, muscles may become stiff or floppy, making it challenging to move and control arms and legs.

CP affects each person differently. Some children may struggle with walking, while others may have difficulty speaking clearly.

Despite the challenges CP presents, there are ways to help children thrive. While there is no cure for CP, therapy such as stretching exercises and practice can improve movement and muscle control. Additionally, various tools and technologies, such as special walkers, braces, and computer programs, can simplify everyday tasks.

Symptoms

Every child with CP is unique, but some things might be a bit trickier for them. Their muscles might be too stiff (like a board) or too floppy (like a ragdoll), making it harder to crawl, walk, or hold things. Their movements might be jerky or wobbly, as if they are trying to catch butterflies with their hands. Sometimes, they might have trouble speaking clearly, or their voice might sound different. Some children with CP might drool more than others or have trouble swallowing, leading to increased fatigue as their bodies work harder.

Additionally, some children with CP may experience difficulty learning new things, remembering, or paying attention. It is as if there is a little bit of static on the line between the brain and the body. However, not all children with CP face these challenges, and it can vary greatly among individuals. Some kids might simply need a bit more time to understand things, while others might get frustrated easily.

These challenges do not indicate a lack of intelligence in your child. Their brain simply works in a different way. Perhaps they excel at puzzles or have a great memory for faces. By focusing on your child's strengths, you can find ways to help them overcome obstacles. Special teaching methods and tools can make learning easier and more enjoyable. Additionally, therapists are available to assist children with CP in developing their skills.

Variations in Severity - Mild, Moderate, and Severe

Think of CP like a spectrum, akin to the colors of a rainbow. On one end, the challenges are milder, while on the other, they are more significant. Some children with CP may walk a little unevenly but can get around just fine without needing any special equipment. Others might require assistance with walking, using braces or a walker for increased mobility. In more severe cases, a child might rely on a wheelchair for mobility.

The severity of CP does not necessarily dictate the future. With therapy and support, a child's abilities can improve over time. Each child is unique; even those with similar CP diagnoses may exhibit different strengths and weaknesses. It is essential to focus on the possibilities and reassure parents that therapies and tools are available to help their child reach their full potential, regardless of the severity of their condition.

Impact on Daily Life Activities

CP can make some everyday tasks a little trickier. Getting dressed, brushing teeth, or playing with toys may be challenging due to muscle stiffness or weakness. Imagine trying to button a shirt with mittens on; that is kind of what it can be like when muscles are stiff or floppy.

Therapists can be likened to personal trainers; they teach exercises and strategies to help your child move their body in the best way possible. Tools act as helpers; special spoons, cups, or adapted toys can make everyday tasks easier. Since every child's needs are different, discuss how therapies and tools can be customized to address their specific challenges.

Just like everyone has their own style, your child will find ways to do things that work for them. It might take a little longer, but they will get there. Focus on what the child can do, highlight their strengths, and celebrate their progress, no matter how small. Independence is key. As much as possible, encourage the child to do things themselves, even if it takes extra time or patience. With support and the right tools, your child can still live a full and happy life.

Different Types of Cerebral Palsy

Imagine the brain as a big control center, sending messages to different parts of the body to move. In CP, there is a mix-up in these messages, but it can affect different parts of the body in various ways. This is why there are a few different types.

One type makes muscles stiff (spastic CP), kind of like they are always a little tense, which can make it hard to move arms and legs smoothly. Another type makes movements jerky and uncontrolled (dyskinetic CP). It might feel like trying to write with a shaky hand. There is also a type that affects balance and coordination (ataxic CP), making it wobbly to walk or stand. Many children have a mix of these types (mixed CP).

The type of CP does not necessarily determine the severity. A child with any type of CP can face a range of challenges. Focus on what matters most, helping your child. There are therapies and tools that can improve movement and function, regardless of the specific type.

There are ways to help your child reach their full potential.

Causes of Cerebral Palsy

Imagine the brain as a delicate building site while your baby is growing in the tummy. Sometimes, things can go wrong during this construction process. There are several reasons why the building blocks of the brain might not fit together perfectly. Sometimes, the brain might not receive enough oxygen or blood flow, which can occur before birth, during birth, or shortly after. An infection the mother contracts during pregnancy can sometimes reach the baby and affect the brain's development. In rare cases, there might be a problem with the baby's genes. It is important to know that in many cases, doctors cannot pinpoint the exact cause of CP.

The factors we mentioned are not the parents' fault, and there is usually nothing that could have been prevented. Focus on what you can control now.

Diagnosis of Cerebral Palsy

Imagine your child's development is like a race. There are milestones most children reach at certain ages, such as rolling over, sitting up, and walking. Doctors closely monitor these milestones. If there appears to be a delay, they might suspect CP.

To diagnose CP, doctors typically undertake several steps. They ask you questions about your child's birth and medical history, conduct a physical exam to assess muscle tone, reflexes, and movement, and may recommend tests like brain scans to check for any signs of brain damage.

It is important to understand that diagnosing CP can take time. There is not a single test, and doctors want to be certain before making a diagnosis.

An early diagnosis is crucial. The sooner therapy and support can commence, the better the outcome for your child. If you have any concerns about your child's development, do not hesitate to talk to your doctor. Ask questions and express your worries.

Remember to be patient and understanding, as most parents are likely to have many questions and emotions during the diagnosis process.

2. LIVING WITH CEREBRAL PALSY

Common Medical Concerns

Because CP affects the brain's messages to the body, it can sometimes lead to other issues. Some children with CP might experience difficulty swallowing or chewing, making eating challenging and frustrating. Fortunately, there are special tools and exercises available to help with this.

Additionally, muscles that are too stiff (spastic) can hinder deep breathing, necessitating regular chest physiotherapy.

Sometimes, the brain glitch in CP can also affect other areas, potentially resulting in seizures or vision and hearing problems. It is important to monitor for these issues and address them promptly if necessary. Moreover, growing bones and muscles can become misaligned when they are not moving enough, underscoring the importance of regular check-ups with a doctor to monitor growth and prevent problems.

These concerns are common and manageable, with specialists and therapies available to address each issue. The focus is on prevention, with regular doctor visits and therapy aiding in identifying and addressing potential problems early on.

Imagine your child's brain as a coach, and their muscles as the players. Therapy serves as practice sessions that help the coach and players work together better. With CP, the messages between the brain and muscles can become mixed up. Therapy exercises help clarify these messages from the brain and enable the muscles to respond more effectively. Just like any sport, practice makes perfect. Therapy aids in strengthening your child's muscles, enhancing flexibility, and improving coordination. This, in turn, makes it easier for them to perform activities such as walking, crawling, or using a wheelchair more easily, speaking more clearly, engaging in play with toys and interacting with others, and taking care of themselves as they grow older.

Different types of therapy

- **Physical therapy:** Helps with movement, strength, and balance.
- **Occupational therapy:** Teaches daily living skills like dressing, eating, and playing.
- **Speech therapy:** Helps with communication and speaking clearly.

Therapy is most effective when started early. The brain is more adaptable in young children, so early intervention can make a big difference. Therapy is a journey, not a quick fix. It takes time and consistent effort to see results, but the benefits are long-lasting. Therapy can have a positive impact on the child's life. It is an investment in their future independence and well-being.

Role of Therapy in Daily Life

Communication: Imagine talking is like a team sport. Your brain sends messages to your mouth, tongue, and voice box to produce sounds and words. In CP, this team might not always be perfectly coordinated, making speaking clearly difficult for some children. There are many ways to communicate, not just through talking. Pictures, gestures, and even special devices can assist children with CP in expressing themselves. Therapists can aid children in developing their communication skills. They can teach them new ways to express themselves and help them practice speaking more clearly.

Development: Every child develops at their own pace, and that is okay. Some children with CP might reach milestones like walking or talking a little later than others. CP can sometimes affect muscle control, which in turn can impact development. This might make it harder for a child to reach for toys or roll over at first. Fortunately, there are many therapies available to help children with CP reach their developmental milestones. These therapies can strengthen muscles, improve coordination, and support overall development.

Focus on progress, not perfection. Celebrate even small improvements in communication and development. Every child is unique. Some children with CP might experience developmental delays in one area but excel in another. Early intervention is key. The sooner a child starts therapy, the better their chances of reaching their full potential.

Emotional and Social Development

Just like everyone else, children with CP experience feelings like happiness, sadness, and frustration. Sometimes, due to CP, it can be harder for them to express their feelings. They might get frustrated if they cannot move the way they want to, which can lead to meltdowns or tears. Playing with other children is super important for everyone, but it might be trickier for children with CP. They might need a little extra help joining in activities or communicating their needs.

The good news is there are ways to help. Therapists can teach children healthy ways to express their emotions. Social play is still possible. There are adapted games and activities that everyone can enjoy. Parents are key. You can help your child by talking about emotions, using picture cards, and encouraging interaction with other children. Even though there might be challenges, your child can still develop healthy emotions and strong social connections.

3. FOSTERING INDEPENDENCE

Setting Realistic Goals

Imagine goals as stepping stones across a river. We want to help your child reach the other side, but taking giant leaps can be frustrating. Smaller, achievable goals are like stepping stones closer together. They help your child build confidence and celebrate successes along the way.

For example, instead of aiming to walk a mile right away, maybe we start with walking across the room. As your child gets stronger, we can gradually increase the distance.

Set goals together with your child (if age-appropriate). Ask them what they would like to be able to do, and work together to break it down into smaller steps.

Focus on what your child can do, not what they cannot. This helps build a positive and motivating atmosphere. Celebrate every step of the way. Even small achievements deserve recognition.

Therapists can be a great help. They can assess your child's abilities and recommend goals that are both challenging and achievable. Remember, the key is to be encouraging and focus on progress, not perfection. Small wins lead to big accomplishments.

Building Self-Esteem

Self-esteem is how good we feel about ourselves. It is like a superhero cape that helps us face challenges. Children with CP might encounter some things that make it harder to feel good about themselves. Maybe it is because moving around is tricky, or perhaps because things take a little longer. The good news is there are ways to help your child feel like a superhero.

Focus on what they can do. Celebrate their achievements, no matter how small. Did they finally master putting on their shoes? Did they speak up in class? Make a big deal about it. Let them try new things. Even if it takes some practice, encourage them to explore their interests, like sports, art, or music. There are often ways to adapt activities for them to participate. Be their biggest cheerleader. Offer encouragement and support when things get tough. Let them know you believe in them, even when they get frustrated. Help them find their tribe. Connect them with other kids who face similar challenges. Having friends who understand can be a huge boost to self-esteem.

Be patient. Building self-esteem takes time and effort. Focus on effort, not just the outcome. Praise your child for trying hard, even if they do not achieve perfection. Be a role model. Show your child that you accept yourself, flaws, and all. By following these tips, parents can help their child with CP develop a strong sense of self-worth and feel like the superhero they truly are.

Encouraging Exploration and Play

Play is super important for all kids, even those with CP. It is how they learn, grow, and have fun. Think of play as a workout for the brain and body; it helps them develop new skills like reaching, grasping, and moving around. Even if your child cannot move exactly like other kids, there are ways they can explore and play.

Make playtime fun and engaging. Choose toys with bright colors, interesting textures, and sounds. Get down on their level. Floor time is great for exploration and helps with reaching and grasping. Think outside the box. Use everyday objects for play. Scarves can become capes, pots and pans become drums. Focus on what they can do. If reaching is difficult, use toys with big buttons or handles. Make it a team effort. Play with your child and their siblings. This helps with social interaction and communication.

Be patient. It might take a little longer for your child to explore, but that does not mean they are not learning. Celebrate every accomplishment. No matter how small, praise your child's efforts to explore and play. There are also therapists who can help. Occupational therapists can suggest specific activities and adaptations to make play more accessible for your child. By focusing on fun and celebrating their child's unique abilities, parents can create a world of exploration and play for their child with CP.

Adaptive Equipment and Technology

Imagine there are tools that can help your child do things a little easier. These are called adaptive equipment and technology. Think of them as special helpers. Just like we might use a spoon to eat soup, adaptive equipment can make everyday tasks like dressing, getting around, or playing more manageable.

There are many different types of helpers. These helpers can make your child feel more independent and confident. They can also help them participate in activities they might find challenging otherwise.

- **For moving around:** Walkers, wheelchairs, braces, standing frames (helps them practice standing), leg lifters (helps get legs into chairs or beds).
- **For daily activities:** Special utensils, weighted vests (feels calming and helps focus), buttons with loops for easier grabbing, dressing sticks (long grabber to help put on socks), bathroom equipment.
- **For communication:** Picture boards with symbols to point to what they want, voice synthesizers (speaks what they type), eye-tracking computers (controlled by eye movements), special keyboards, trackpads with joysticks, voice recognition software.

Not every child will need all the helpers. A therapist can assess your child's needs and recommend the most suitable equipment.

Technology is always improving. There are cool things like apps that can help with communication or games that are accessible for everyone. Focus on the benefits. Let the parents know that adaptive equipment is there to empower their child and help them reach their full potential.

Adaptive equipment is about helping the child be as independent as possible, and there is no shame in using these tools. Imagine there are tools that can help your child do things a little easier. Adaptive equipment is not one-size-fits-all. The therapist will work with you to find the tools that best suit your child's needs. Technology is constantly evolving. There are new and exciting tools being developed all the time to help children with CP. Focus on independence. Adaptive equipment can help your child become more independent and do things for themselves, which can boost their confidence. These tools can empower their child and help them reach their full potential.

4. EDUCATION AND ADVOCACY

Finding the Right Educational Setting

The educational journey for a child with Cerebral Palsy (CP) requires careful consideration. This section explores two key areas of decision-making: Public Schools vs. Specialized Programs, and Inclusion and Least Restrictive Environment (LRE) with a focus on Individual Needs and Learning Styles.

Public Schools vs. Specialized Programs

The choice between public schools and specialized programs hinges on a child's specific needs:

- **Public Schools:** Public schools offer a diverse learning environment with opportunities for socialization and exposure to various subjects. These schools are mandated by law to provide an Inclusive Least Restrictive Environment (LRE) and can offer Individualized Education Programs (IEPs) for additional support.
- **Specialized Programs:** These programs cater specifically to children with disabilities, offering specialized instruction and a high teacher-to-student ratio. However, opportunities for interaction with typically developing peers might be limited.

Collaboration is Key

The ideal educational setting fosters inclusion and development:

- **Inclusion and Least Restrictive Environment (LRE):** The legal framework prioritizes placing children with CP in regular classrooms with their peers, promoting social interaction and skill development.

- **Individualized Education Programs (IEPs):** IEPs provide tailored support for each child, potentially including specialized materials, therapy sessions, or curriculum adjustments.
- **Collaborative Efforts:** Educators receive training to effectively support students with CP, while open communication between parents and teachers ensures ongoing collaboration and problem-solving.

Understanding the Individual

A child's unique learning style and needs are paramount:

- **Understanding Individual Needs:** Children with CP may face challenges with mobility, coordination, communication, or cognitive processing. Needs can range from physical assistance to specialized furniture or alternative communication methods.
- **Identifying Learning Styles:** Understanding a child's preferred learning style, whether visual, auditory, kinesthetic, or tactile, allows for adapting teaching methods and utilizing assistive technology to maximize learning potential.
- **Collaboration with Teachers and Therapists:** Open communication with teachers and therapists allows for the development of strategies and accommodations to meet a child's specific needs and learning style.

The educational journey for a child with CP requires a multi-faceted approach. By carefully considering the options of public schools vs. specialized programs, embracing the principles of inclusion and LRE, and prioritizing a child's individual needs and learning styles, parents, educators, and therapists can work together to create a supportive and enriching educational environment that fosters academic success, social development, and a lasting love of learning.

Working with Teachers and Therapists

This section explores the importance of collaboration with teachers and therapists, focusing on effective communication and collaboration, developing an Individualized Education Program (IEP), and understanding 504 Plans and accommodations.

The Power of Teamwork

A strong support system is vital for a child with CP to thrive.

- **Effective Communication:** Regular meetings with teachers and therapists facilitate information sharing, address concerns, and ensure everyone understands the child's needs.
- **Open Collaboration:** Openness and honesty ensure a collaborative approach. Setting common goals and celebrating achievements together fosters a supportive environment.
- **Sharing Expertise:** Teachers and therapists bring unique expertise to the table. Collaborative discussions ensure a consistent approach to the child's development.
- **Respecting Each Other:** Building a strong team involves getting to know everyone involved and treating them with respect.
- **Advocacy for Your Child:** As your child's advocate, you ensure they receive the necessary support to thrive in school.

Understanding IEPs and 504 Plans

The educational journey for a child with Cerebral Palsy (CP) requires a tailored approach. This section explores Individualized Education Programs (IEPs) and 504 Plans, highlighting their components, benefits, and the importance of advocating for your child's needs.

Individualized Education Program (IEP)

An IEP serves as a personalized roadmap for a child with CP's educational journey and success.

- **Present Levels of Academic Achievement and Functional Performance (PLAAFP):** This section assesses the child's current skills and how CP impacts their learning.
- **Annual Goals:** Clear and measurable goals are established, targeting academic progress or independent living skills.
- **Special Education and Related Services:** This outlines the specific support the child needs, such as therapy services or specialized instruction.
- **Supplementary Aids and Services:** Modifications to the learning environment or classroom activities are detailed here, ensuring accessibility and success.
- **Progress Monitoring:** Regular evaluations track the child's progress and ensure the IEP remains effective.
- **Transition Services:** For older students, this plan outlines future plans towards college, vocational training, or independent living.

Developing the IEP is a collaborative effort

Parents, teachers, therapists, and the child (when age-appropriate) work together to create and update the IEP, ensuring it adapts to the child's evolving needs.

- **The Support Team:** Teachers, therapists, and parents collaborate to create the IEP.
- **Understanding the Child:** The team evaluates the child's strengths, weaknesses, learning style, and CP-related needs.
- **Setting Goals:** Clear and achievable academic and CP-related goals are established.
- **Providing Support:** The IEP details the specific support the child needs, including modifications, accommodations, and related services.

- **Regular Communication:** IEP meetings and ongoing communication between parents, teachers, and therapists ensure the child's needs are met consistently.
- **Advocacy and Collaboration:** Parents actively participate in IEP meetings, sharing observations and concerns, to create the best possible learning environment.

Empowering Participation with 504 Plans

A 504 Plan equips children with CP to participate fully in the general education setting.

- **Equal Opportunities:** This plan ensures children with CP have access to the same learning opportunities and activities as their peers, fostering inclusion.
- **Accommodations:** The plan outlines specific accommodations, such as extra time on tests, assistive technology, or preferential seating, to remove barriers to learning.
- **Rights and Protections:** 504 Plans ensure children with CP have access to a free and appropriate public education, protection from discrimination, and privacy regarding their disability.

Obtaining a 504 Plan

Parents should consult their child's doctor or teacher to initiate the process of creating a 504 Plan with school administrators.

Leveling the Playing Field with 504 Plan

A 504 Plan is basically a roadmap for how a school can support a child with a disability in a regular classroom setting. It is named after Section 504 of the Rehabilitation Act, a law that prevents discrimination against people with disabilities (USA).

- **Goal:** Level the playing field and give the child with a disability an equal chance to learn alongside their peers.
- **Who it is for:** Students with disabilities that do not require special education but still need some accommodations to succeed in school. This could include conditions like ADHD, dyslexia, or certain physical limitations.
- **What it includes:**
    - Specific accommodations tailored to the child's individual needs. Examples include extra time on tests, preferential seating, access to audiobooks, or using a computer for written assignments.
    - Strategies to remove any barriers that might be hindering the child's learning.

504 Plans ensure equal access to learning for children with disabilities

- **Purpose of a 504 Plan:** This plan outlines accommodations, like extra time or assistive technology, to help a child with CP learn without changing the learning goals.
- **Initiating the Process:** Consult your child's doctor and teacher to request a 504 Plan meeting with school administrators.
- **Advocacy is Key:** As your child's advocate, share information about their CP and how it affects their learning.
- **Adapting to Change:** 504 Plans can be updated as the child's needs evolve, ensuring continuous support.

Here is a key difference to remember. A 504 Plan is different from an Individualized Education Program (IEP). An IEP is for students with disabilities who require more specialized instruction and support, often outside the regular classroom setting.

Effective communication and collaboration with teachers and therapists are essential for a child with CP to reach their full potential.

Developing an Individualized Education Program and understanding 504 Plans and accommodations empower parents to be active participants in their child's education. By working together, this team can create a supportive and enriching learning environment where a child with CP can flourish.

The US concept of a 504 Plan does not have a direct equivalent in the UK and Australia. However, both countries have similar legislation that aims to provide support for students with disabilities in mainstream education though 'Reasonable adjustments' to prevent discrimination.

The Power of Advocacy

As your child's strongest advocate, you play a crucial role in their education.

- **Understanding Your Child's Needs:** Collaborate with doctors, therapists, and teachers to create a comprehensive understanding of your child's specific learning needs.
- **Communication and Collaboration:** Maintain open communication with school staff, discussing your child's progress and working together on solutions.
- **Knowing Your Rights:** Educate yourself on your child's rights under disability laws, ensuring their needs are met.
- **Positive Reinforcement:** Celebrate your child's progress, fostering confidence and a positive attitude towards learning.
- **Involving Your Child:** As your child matures, involve them in discussions about their education, empowering them to become active participants in their learning journey.

IEPs and 504 Plans are valuable tools to ensure children with CP receive the support they need to thrive in school. By understanding these plans, advocating for your child's needs, and collaborating with educators and therapists, you can guide them towards a fulfilling and successful educational experience.

Parent's Guide to Advocacy

For parents raising a child with Cerebral Palsy (CP), the educational journey requires a champion – you. This section explores the multifaceted role of a parent-advocate, focusing on understanding educational rights, fostering effective communication, and navigating the educational system.

Understanding Your Child's Rights

The Individuals with Disabilities Education Act (IDEA) serves as a legal foundation for educational equity.

- **Free and Appropriate Public Education (FAPE):** IDEA guarantees children with CP the right to attend public schools and receive an education tailored to their individual needs.
- **Individualized Education Programs (IEPs):** IEPs are customized plans outlining a child's specific needs, goals, and required support services.
- **Parental Rights and Participation:** Parents have the right to participate in IEP meetings, request evaluations, and advocate for any necessary revisions.

Knowing your child's rights empowers you to become a strong advocate for their educational success. Many resources, like disability advocacy groups, can assist you in navigating this process.

Effective Communication with Professionals

Clear and effective communication is vital when collaborating with professionals to ensure your child's needs are met.

- **Preparation and Knowledge:** Observe and document your child's behavior, research CP, and formulate questions about your concerns and goals.
- **Clarity and Structure:** Start with the basics, use simple language, and be specific about your child's needs during appointments.
- **Active Listening and Advocacy:** Actively listen to professionals' advice, ask clarifying questions, express concerns, and advocate for your child's well-being.
- **Support Strategies:** Consider bringing a support person, utilizing technology (like recording conversations), and confidently advocating for your child.

By fostering strong and open communication, you can work collaboratively with professionals to develop a comprehensive support system for your child.

A Collaborative Approach

Informed decisions and collaboration with school teams are essential for a child with CP's educational journey.

- **Least Restrictive Environment (LRE):** The legal framework emphasizes placing children with CP in inclusive settings (LRE) alongside their peers whenever possible.
- **Understanding School Options:** Public schools offer inclusive environments, while specialized programs cater specifically to children with disabilities. The best choice depends on your child's individual needs.
- **Individualized Education Programs (IEPs):** IEPs are legal documents outlining your child's unique needs, including accommodations, modifications, or related services (therapy).
- **Seeking Support:** Numerous organizations offer resources, guidance, and support to parents navigating the educational system for children with disabilities.

Becoming your child's advocate is an empowering and crucial role. With knowledge, strong communication skills, and a collaborative approach with the educational system, you can champion your child's educational success.

Remember, you are not alone. There are resources and a community of support ready to help you navigate this journey.

5. BUILDING A SUPPORT SYSTEM

The Importance of Family Support

Cerebral Palsy (CP) presents a unique set of challenges for children and their families. However, the unwavering support of a loving family unit serves as a cornerstone for a child with CP to navigate life with confidence and resilience.

This section explores the significance of open communication, shared responsibilities within the family, and building resilience as a whole.

Open Communication & Shared Responsibilities

Open communication fosters a foundation of understanding and collaboration within the family.

- **Understanding Each Other's Needs:** Open communication allows family members to voice their needs and concerns, fostering empathy and creating a more supportive environment.
- **Collaborative Decision-Making:** Joint decision-making empowers children with CP and strengthens family bonds.
- **Building Confidence:** Open communication promotes a sense of security and self-worth in the child with CP.
- **Managing Stress:** Sharing concerns and challenges helps to alleviate stress and promotes effective problem-solving.
- **Sharing Responsibilities:** Distributing responsibilities among family members lightens the burden and allows everyone to contribute.
- **Building a Support Network:** Seeking support from extended family, friends, and support groups strengthens the family unit and provides additional resources.

Supporting Siblings & Family Members

The presence of CP within a family can impact all members.

- **Addressing Sibling Needs:** Acknowledge the unique challenges and emotions siblings may experience. Create a safe space for open communication and address feelings of frustration or jealousy.
- **Strategies for Sibling Support:** Provide age-appropriate explanations of CP, encourage independence in siblings while fostering quality time together, and connect siblings with support groups.
- **Supporting Extended Family:** Educate other family members about CP and its implications. Prioritize self-care for parents to maintain their well-being. Seek additional support from therapists or support groups if needed.
- **Fostering a Supportive Environment:** Open communication, celebrating differences within the family, and prioritizing support for all members foster an inclusive and loving environment where everyone thrives.

Building Resilience as a Family

Navigating CP requires a collective effort of resilience and positive thinking.

- **Understanding CP:** Knowledge is power. Openly discuss CP, address anxieties, and research available resources.
- **Focusing on Strengths:** Celebrate the child's unique abilities and talents, fostering a sense of self-worth.
- **Shared Involvement:** Involve all family members in the child's care, creating a sense of shared responsibility and connection.
- **Prioritizing Self-Care:** Taking time for self-care allows parents to recharge and maintain their ability to support their child.

- **Celebrating Achievements:** Recognize and celebrate all achievements, both big and small, to build confidence and motivation.
- **Seeking Help When Needed:** Do not hesitate to seek assistance from professionals or support groups. Remember, resilience is a journey, not a destination.
- **Maintaining Positivity:** A positive outlook strengthens the family unit and fosters a hopeful future for the child with CP.

The unwavering support of a loving family plays a vital role in the life of a child with CP. By fostering open communication, sharing responsibilities, and building resilience as a family unit, families can create a supportive environment where children with CP can thrive and reach their full potential.

Remember, collaboration, understanding, and a positive outlook are key ingredients for building a hopeful future for children with CP and their families.

Connecting with Other Parents

This section explores the importance of connecting with other parents of children with CP, highlighting the benefits of online communities, sharing experiences and advice, and finding strength and inspiration from others.

Support Network of Online Communities

The internet offers a wealth of resources and a sense of belonging.

- **Online Communities and Support Groups:** Seek out online communities and support groups specifically for parents of children with CP. These connections foster a sense of belonging and offer invaluable resources.

- **Benefits of Online Support:** These groups provide valuable information on therapies, resources, and emotional support during difficult times.
- **Finding the Right Community:** Utilize social media platforms, CP organization websites, or search engines to locate these online communities.
- **Responsible Online Communication:** Maintain respectful communication, share your experiences thoughtfully, and prioritize privacy when engaging online.
- **Combining Online and Local Support:** Complement online connections by joining local support groups for deeper in-person connections.

The Value of Shared Experiences

Connecting with others who understand your journey fosters a sense of community.

- **Emotional Support and Shared Understanding:** Sharing experiences with parents facing similar challenges offers comfort, empathy, and practical advice.
- **Finding Common Ground and Support:** Support groups, online communities, parent-teacher conferences, and therapy sessions provide opportunities to connect with other parents.
- **Open Communication and Respectful Exchange:** Embrace open communication, offer support to others, respect diverse experiences, and celebrate each other's successes.

Finding Strength and Inspiration

Connecting with others empowers you on the journey of raising your child with CP.

- **Strength in Numbers:** Knowing you're not alone and sharing experiences can be a source of strength and resilience.
- **Inspiration from Others' Successes:** Be inspired by the stories and accomplishments of other parents and their children with CP.
- **Finding Support Through Shared Experiences:** Support groups, online communities, and events focused on CP provide opportunities to connect with others who understand.
- **Openness, Compassion, and Celebrating Success:** Approach interactions with openness, listen attentively to others' experiences, respect diverse approaches, and celebrate each other's successes.
- **A Community of Support:** Remember, there is a whole community of parents cheering you and your child on.

Connecting with other parents of children with CP is an invaluable resource. By building a network of support through online communities and local groups, sharing experiences and advice, and finding strength in shared goals, you can build a supportive environment for your child to thrive. Remember, you are not alone on this journey. There is a community of parents ready to offer support, empathy, and inspiration.

Finding Community Resources

For families raising a child with Cerebral Palsy (CP), navigating the complex landscape of support can be daunting.

This section explores three key areas where community resources offer invaluable assistance: Early Intervention Programs, Recreational Activities and Social Opportunities, and Financial Assistance and Government Benefits.

Early Intervention Programs

Early intervention is crucial for maximizing a child's potential with CP.

- **Identifying Resources:** Utilize government websites to find federal and state-level Early Intervention Programs (EIP).
- **Non-Profit Support:** Seek resources and support from non-profit organizations and locate local CP chapters.
- **Collaboration with Professionals:** Your child's doctor, the special education department of your local school district, and children's hospitals can provide information and referrals to EIP services.
- **Taking Action for Your Child:** By actively seeking information and connecting with resources, you can ensure your child receives the support they need to thrive in the early years.

Fostering Social Connections and Recreation

Community resources offer opportunities for social interaction and recreation.

- **Exploring Options:** Consult your child's doctor or therapists for recommendations on local programs catering to children with CP.
- **National Organizations as a Starting Point:** National organizations organize events and camps specifically designed for children with CP.
- **Online Resources:** Search disability resource websites or check your city's parks and recreation department for relevant programs.
- **Adaptive Sports and Activities:** Consider options like wheelchair basketball, or explore local activities at community centers, museums, or libraries that offer accessibility features.
- **Starting Small and Prioritizing Comfort:** Begin with activities that cater to your child's comfort level, gradually expanding their participation as they become more comfortable.

Financial Support & Government Benefits

Financial assistance programs can lessen the financial burden of caring for a child with CP.

- **Seeking Guidance Within Healthcare Systems:** Hospitals or clinics where your child receives treatment may have social workers or resources to help identify local support options.
- **Disability Organizations:** Look for disability organizations in your area specializing in CP, as they often provide workshops or consultations on obtaining benefits.
- **Government Websites:** Research disability services or financial aid programs offered by government agencies through their websites.
- **National Organizations as Information Hubs:** Trusted national organizations provide valuable information on benefits and assistance programs.
- **Considering Legal Expertise:** Seek advice from a disability law specialist for guidance in navigating the application process for benefits and legal protections.
- **Persistence and Utilizing Available Resources:** Financial assistance programs exist to support families caring for children with CP. Be specific in your search, do not hesitate to call for information, and persist in finding the right resources.

Community resources are a vital support system for families raising a child with CP. By seeking out Early Intervention Programs, exploring Recreational Activities and Social Opportunities, and navigating Financial Assistance and Government Benefits, families can create a supportive environment that fosters their child's growth and development.

Remember, collaboration with professionals, persistence in seeking resources, and a commitment to your child's well-being are key ingredients for building a bright future for your child with CP.

Taking Care of Yourself

Raising a child with Cerebral Palsy (CP) is a journey filled with love and immense challenges. The demands of caregiving can leave parents feeling depleted. This section explores the importance of self-care for parents of children with CP, emphasizing the need to balance their own needs with those of their child, and identifying resources for stress management and support.

Self-Care Matters

Prioritizing self-care is not a luxury for parents of children with CP; it is a necessity.

- **Maintaining Physical Health:** Regular checkups, healthy eating, adequate sleep, and exercise form the foundation for a resilient caregiver.
- **Nurturing Emotional Well-being:** Relaxation techniques like meditation, seeking support from loved ones, and setting boundaries are essential for emotional well-being.
- **Embracing Respite:** Respite care, short breaks, and delegating tasks allow for moments of rejuvenation and prevent burnout.
- **Self-care is Not Selfish:** By prioritizing self-care, parents are better equipped to be the loving and supportive caregivers their children with CP need.
- **Additional Resources:** Organizations like The Family Caregiver Alliance and The Arc offer tailored support for parents of children with special needs.

Finding Balance

Creating a balance between your child's needs and your own is key.

- **Schedule Time for Yourself:** Carve out time for activities you enjoy, even if it is just a few minutes a day.
- **Seek Help When Needed:** Do not be afraid to ask family, friends, or professionals for help.
- **Prioritize Your Health:** Regular checkups and a healthy lifestyle ensure you can be there for your child in the long run.
- **Connecting with Others:** Support groups allow you to share experiences and find strength in community.
- **Focus on Quality Time:** Engage in activities together, create routines that work for you, and consider respite care when needed.
- **Communication and Collaboration:** Open communication with your partner, therapists, and celebrating achievements all contribute to a balanced approach.

Finding Support and Managing Stress

There are numerous resources available to help you manage stress.

- **Support Groups and Online Communities:** Connect with other parents to share experiences and find common ground.
- **Professional Support:** Therapy or parenting coaching can provide guidance and improve communication within the family.
- **Self-Care Strategies:** Respite care, mindfulness exercises, exercise, hobbies, healthy sleep habits, and relaxation techniques are all effective tools for stress management.
- **Exploring Resources:** Disability organizations, national organizations, and mental health hotlines offer valuable support.
- **Prioritizing Well-Being is Essential:** Taking care of yourself allows you to be the best possible caregiver for your child.

The journey of raising a child with CP requires a resilient caregiver. By prioritizing self-care, striking a balance between needs, and accessing available resources for stress management and support, parents can build a foundation for a fulfilling and enriching life for both themselves and their child with CP.

Remember, you are not alone. There are resources and a community of support ready to help you navigate this journey.

6. PREPARING FOR THE FUTURE

Transitioning to Adulthood

The transition from carefree youth to responsible adulthood is a significant milestone for everyone, and young adults with Cerebral Palsy (CP) are no exception.

This section explores the importance of planning and early preparation, focusing on educational and vocational options, and acquiring independent living skills, to empower young adults with CP to navigate this transition with confidence and independence.

Educational and Vocational Options

Early exploration of educational and vocational opportunities is crucial.

- **Individualized Transition Plans (ITP):** Schools play a vital role by developing ITPs in collaboration with students and families. These plans explore goals, strengths, and interests to identify suitable educational pathways.
- **Focus on Abilities and Interests:** Guiding young adults towards educational paths that capitalize on their strengths and interests is essential. This could involve colleges, vocational training programs, or specialized programs catering to their unique needs.
- **Beyond Education: Vocational Support:** Support services like vocational rehabilitation or supported employment programs can equip young adults with CP with job-specific skills and assist them in finding suitable employment opportunities.
- **Accessibility and Technology:** Ensuring educational institutions and workplaces are accessible is paramount. Exploring

assistive technologies can further empower young adults with CP to succeed in their chosen fields.

Building Independence

Developing strong independent living skills fosters self-reliance and confidence.

- **Occupational Therapy and Life Skills Programs:** Occupational therapy and life skills programs equip young adults with CP with the necessary skills to manage daily tasks, such as personal care, financial management, and household chores.
- **Integration into Educational Planning:** Incorporating independent living skills development into educational plans ensures a holistic approach to preparing young adults for adulthood.
- **Leveraging Technology for Daily Living:** Investigating and utilizing assistive technologies can significantly improve a young adult's ability to perform daily tasks independently.
- **Individualized Support and Celebrating Progress:** Every person with CP has unique needs. It is crucial to listen to their aspirations, celebrate their achievements, and tailor the support system accordingly.

Planning for a Smooth Transition

Starting the preparation process early paves the way for a more seamless transition.

- **Life Skills Development and Healthcare Management:** Teaching young adults with CP essential life skills like self-care, financial management, and basic healthcare management empowers them to take charge of their lives.

- **Exploring Educational and Vocational Options:** Early exploration of educational and vocational opportunities allows for informed decisions and a smoother transition into the workforce.
- **Decision-Making Skills and Responsibility:** Gradually increasing responsibilities empowers young adults with CP to make independent decisions and fosters confidence in their abilities.
- **Planning for Future Needs:** Addressing future needs such as housing options, transportation solutions, and potential support services ensures a well-rounded plan for a fulfilling adult life.

Transitioning to adulthood with CP presents unique challenges, but with early planning, a focus on educational and vocational opportunities, and the development of independent living skills, young adults with CP can navigate this phase with confidence and lay the foundation for a successful and fulfilling future.

Remember, support, early preparation, and a focus on individual strengths are key ingredients for a smooth and empowering transition into adulthood.

Career Options and Independent Living

The transition to adulthood for young adults with Cerebral Palsy (CP) presents both challenges and exciting possibilities.

This section explores strategies to help them navigate this transition, focusing on exploring career options, promoting supported employment and community integration, and fostering independence in daily life.

Discovering Passions and Building Skills

Finding a fulfilling career is key to independence and self-esteem.

- **Self-Discovery and Exploration:** Encourage young adults with CP to identify their interests and strengths. Discuss potential career paths, acknowledging any challenges related to CP.
- **Experiential Learning:** Facilitate exploration through programs offering job shadowing, internships, or career fairs for individuals with disabilities. These experiences provide valuable insights into potential career paths.
- **Utilizing Online Resources:** Utilize online resources and disability organization websites to research career options and accessibility considerations for various professions.
- **Building a Strong Resume and Portfolio:** Help them craft a resume that showcases their skills and achievements. For creative fields, consider developing a portfolio to highlight their talents.
- **Empowerment and Support:** Remember, the goal is to help them find a career they are passionate about, fostering independence and happiness.

Supported Employment and Community Integration

Supported employment programs create a supportive framework for career exploration and job placement.

- **Identifying Strengths and Interests:** Encourage exploration of hobbies, activities, and assessments to identify potential career paths.
- **Supported Employment Programs:** Investigate and utilize supported employment programs that offer job training, ongoing support, and employer collaboration.
- **Learning Through Observation:** Facilitate job shadowing opportunities and informational interviews to gain firsthand knowledge of different professions.
- **Focus on Abilities:** Shift the focus from limitations to strengths, exploring careers promoting community integration and leveraging their unique talents.

- **Resource Collaboration:** Work with disability organizations, government agencies, and online platforms to access comprehensive career resources and guidance.

Building Confidence and Independence

Encouraging independence in daily activities fosters confidence and self-reliance.

- **Exploration and Skill Development:** Support their exploration of hobbies and activities, fostering a sense of self-discovery and skill development.
- **Identifying Strengths and Interests:** Openly discuss their interests, and consider assessments to identify areas of strength and potential career paths.
- **Matching Skills and Careers:** Research and identify jobs that align with their interests and skillset, focusing on what they can do well.
- **Educational and Training Opportunities:** Explore educational programs or training opportunities that hone the skills needed for their chosen career path.
- **Supportive and Accessible Workplaces:** Seek workplaces that recognize their abilities and are committed to providing necessary accommodations.

Transitioning to adulthood with CP is a journey of self-discovery and empowerment. By exploring career options through experiential learning and supported employment programs, and fostering independence in daily living, young adults with CP can navigate this pivotal phase with confidence and lay the foundation for a fulfilling and independent future.

Remember, collaboration, support, and focusing on individual strengths are key ingredients for success.

Financial Planning and Benefits

Financial planning is crucial for ensuring the well-being of adults with Cerebral Palsy (CP).

This section explores government programs and benefits, educational funding options, and long-term financial security strategies to empower young adults with CP to lead fulfilling and financially secure lives.

Government Programs and Benefits

Government programs offer essential support for adults with CP.

- **Social Security and Medical Benefits:** Gain a comprehensive understanding of programs like Social Security Disability Insurance (SSDI), Supplemental Security Income (SSI), Medicaid, and Medicare. These programs provide vital financial and healthcare support.
- **Seeking Professional Guidance:** Consult with financial advisors specializing in disabilities for personalized advice on navigating these programs effectively.
- **Advocacy and Support Networks:** Empower yourself by learning about your child's rights and connect with other parents of children with CP. Support groups and online resources can offer valuable insights and emotional support.
- **Building a Comprehensive Plan:** Develop a long-term financial plan encompassing healthcare costs, housing, education, and other expenses. This plan ensures their financial well-being throughout their life.

Investing in Education

Planning for educational opportunities is key to a secure future.

- **Individualized Education Programs (IEP):** Utilize the information within your child's IEP to identify and leverage available funding options for educational pursuits.
- **Financial Aid Resources:** Explore federal and state grants, scholarships, and vocational rehabilitation services for financial assistance.
- **Saving for the Future:** Consider establishing a trust fund, a tax-advantaged savings account specifically designed for individuals with disabilities.
- **Employment and Benefits:** Encourage your child to seek employment with benefits packages, and explore additional support programs.
- **Collaboration with Experts:** Connect with disability organizations, financial advisors, and benefits counselors for personalized guidance.
- **Recordkeeping and Advocacy:** Maintain detailed records of your child's needs and progress. Be their advocate and champion their rights throughout the educational journey.

Securing Long-Term Financial Security

Planning for the future ensures your child with CP has a secure foundation.

- **Needs Assessment:** Start by understanding your child's specific needs, encompassing potential government benefits, healthcare costs, and independent living expenses.
- **Early Savings and Risk Management:** Begin saving early to build a financial buffer. Consider life insurance and special needs trusts to safeguard your child's future.
- **Scholarships and Grants:** Research scholarship and grant opportunities to ease the financial burden of higher education or vocational training.

- **Government Support Programs:** Investigate additional financial support available through programs like Social Security Disability Insurance (SSDI).
- **Estate Planning and Guardianship:** Address future considerations through estate planning and explore guardianship options to ensure your child's continued well-being after you are gone.
- **Open Communication and Professional Guidance:** Maintain open communication with your child about their financial needs and goals. Seek guidance from financial advisors and stay informed about community resources available to support families with children with CP.

Financial planning empowers adults with CP to navigate life with confidence. By understanding government programs and benefits, exploring educational funding options, and implementing long-term financial security strategies, you can equip your child with the tools they need to achieve independence, pursue their goals, and live a fulfilling life.

Remember, proactive planning, collaboration with professionals, and unwavering support are key ingredients for a secure and prosperous future.

Building a Hopeful Future

Cerebral Palsy (CP) presents unique challenges, but with careful planning and unwavering support, young adults with CP can build a hopeful and fulfilling future.

This section explores the importance of setting realistic goals, focusing on strengths and abilities, and fostering a vision of independence to empower young adults with CP on their journey to adulthood.

Setting Realistic Goals

Goal setting serves as a roadmap for navigating the path to adulthood.

- **Collaborative Planning:** Engage young adults with CP in discussions about their aspirations. Work together to translate these aspirations into achievable and measurable goals.
- **Focus on Strengths and Interests:** Prioritize goals that capitalize on their strengths and interests, fostering a sense of accomplishment and boosting self-esteem.
- **Breaking Down Big Dreams:** Divide large, long-term dreams into smaller, more manageable steps. This creates a sense of progress and celebrates achievements along the way.
- **Examples of Realistic Goals:** Examples of realistic goals could include learning to cook independently, securing a meaningful job, building friendships, or maintaining good health habits.

Empowerment Through Recognizing Strengths

Focusing on a young adult's strengths fosters confidence and self-belief.

- **Strengths-Based Approach:** Shift the focus from limitations to strengths. Identify their unique talents and celebrate their achievements in everyday tasks.
- **Aligning Goals with Strengths:** Set goals that align with their existing skillset, building confidence and fostering a sense of self-efficacy.
- **Nurturing Interests and Passions:** Support and encourage their interests and passions, fostering personal growth and potential career paths.
- **Collaboration with Professionals:** Work collaboratively with therapists and educators to leverage their expertise and develop a comprehensive support system.

- **Building Confidence for the Future:** Recognizing and building on their strengths equips young adults with CP with the confidence to navigate challenges and pursue their goals.

Envisioning a Fulfilling and Independent Life

Positive visualization fosters hope and motivation.

- **Exploring New Avenues:** Encourage them to explore new activities and hobbies, such as art, sports, or volunteering.
- **Celebrating Accomplishments:** Celebrate successes, big or small, to reinforce positive behaviors and build momentum.
- **Promoting Independence:** Encourage them to make decisions for themselves and advocate for their needs, fostering self-reliance and independence.
- **Leveraging Technology:** Explore assistive technologies that can enhance their independence and daily living skills.
- **Envisioning a Bright Future:** Work together to envision a future where they have a fulfilling job, live independently in a suitable environment, and enjoy meaningful relationships.

Transitioning to adulthood with CP is a journey of self-discovery and empowerment. By setting realistic goals, focusing on strengths and abilities, and envisioning a fulfilling and independent life, young adults with CP can navigate this transition with confidence and optimism.

Remember, collaboration, support, and focusing on individual potential are key ingredients for building a hopeful future. In the United States, organizations like The Cerebral Palsy Foundation, United Cerebral Palsy (UCP), and The Arc offer support, and similar organizations likely exist in other countries.

7. MANAGING EMOTIONS AND BEHAVIOR

Cerebral Palsy (CP) presents both physical and emotional challenges for children.

This section explores the importance of recognizing signs of anxiety, frustration, and depression, understanding the impact of CP on emotional development, and considering communication difficulties when supporting a child's emotional well-being.

Recognizing Signals of Distress

Early intervention is crucial for addressing emotional challenges.

- **Understanding Emotional Cues:** Children with CP may not always express emotions verbally. Be vigilant for signs of anxiety (excessive worry, sleep issues, irritability), frustration (outbursts, withdrawal), or depression (sadness, loss of interest in activities).
- **Open Communication and Professional Support:** Create a safe space for your child to express their feelings, and seek guidance from doctors or therapists if you notice any concerning changes in behavior or mood.
- **Building Confidence and Support Systems:** Celebrate their achievements, promote positive self-esteem, and utilize available resources to help your child navigate emotional challenges.

The Emotional Impact of CP

CP can influence a child's emotional development.

- **Frustration and Social Challenges:** Physical limitations can lead to frustration and difficulty making friends, potentially impacting self-esteem.

- **Recognizing Behavioral Changes:** Watch for signs like anger outbursts, social withdrawal, or negative self-talk. These can indicate emotional distress.
- **Seeking Professional Support and Advocacy:** If you notice any changes, consult doctors or therapists. Remember, you are not alone. Available resources can support both you and your child.

Communication Difficulties and Emotional Expression

Communication is key to understanding a child's emotional state.

- **Navigating Communication Barriers:** Be patient and adapt your communication style. Use simple language, visuals, and assistive devices if necessary.
- **Focus on Body Language and Nonverbal Cues:** Pay attention to facial expressions and vocal tones to understand their emotions.
- **Celebrating Efforts and Open Communication:** Acknowledge and celebrate any attempt at communication, regardless of the method. Let them know all emotions are valid and encourage open communication.
- **Individuality and Patience:** Every child communicates differently. Be open to learning new ways to connect with yours.

Understanding emotional challenges and fostering open communication are essential for supporting children with CP. By recognizing signs of distress, acknowledging the impact of CP on emotional development, and adapting communication methods, you can create a safe and supportive environment where your child feels understood and empowered to express their emotions.

Remember, ongoing support and professional guidance can make a significant difference in their well-being.

Effective Communication Strategies

Cerebral Palsy (CP) can present challenges with communication, but there are effective strategies to bridge the gap and foster strong connections.

This section explores adapting communication methods, practicing active listening, and using positive language to empower children with CP to express themselves effectively.

Tailoring Communication to Individual Needs

Effective communication starts with understanding your child.

- **Decoding Nonverbal Cues:** Observe how your child uses gestures, facial expressions, or pictures to communicate. Respect their chosen method, whether it is pointing, using assistive devices, or vocalizations.
- **Clarity and Patience:** Speak in short, simple sentences and utilize visuals to enhance understanding. Allow ample time for responses and celebrate each attempt at communication, no matter how small.
- **Collaboration with Therapists:** Work with therapists to identify the most effective communication strategies for your child, fostering their ability to express themselves clearly.

The Power of Active Listening

Active listening goes beyond simply hearing what your child says.

- **Undivided Attention:** Give your child your full attention when they attempt to communicate, eliminating distractions and maintaining eye contact. Use body language to show you're engaged.

- **Decoding Nonverbal Communication:** Pay close attention to facial expressions, body movements, and sounds to understand their emotional state and potential needs.
- **Open Communication and Problem-Solving:** If you're unsure of their message, ask clarifying questions to understand their needs and encourage open communication.

Building Confidence

Positive reinforcement fosters a supportive communication environment.

- **Focusing on Strengths:** Highlight your child's strengths and abilities, shifting the focus away from limitations. Use positive language that empowers them.
- **Encouragement and Celebration:** Encourage them to keep trying, even when communication is challenging. Celebrate every small achievement, boosting their confidence and motivation.
- **Building Self-Esteem:** By using positive language and celebrating their efforts, you help your child feel good about themselves and create a safe space for continued learning and growth.

Communication is a cornerstone of connection. By adapting communication methods to your child's individual needs, practicing active listening, and using positive language, you can create a bridge for understanding and empower your child with CP to express themselves effectively.

Remember, patience, support, and celebrating their efforts are key to fostering a strong and meaningful relationship.

Positive Behavior Support Techniques

Positive behavior support empowers children with Cerebral Palsy (CP) to manage their behavior and navigate their world with confidence.

This section explores three key strategies: identifying triggers and setting clear expectations, utilizing redirection and positive reinforcement, and developing a consistent behavior plan with professionals.

Identifying Triggers and Setting Expectations

Effective behavior management starts with understanding the underlying causes.

- **Decoding Triggers:** Collaborate with therapists to identify triggers for challenging behaviors. These could be sensory overload, communication difficulties, or frustration.
- **Clear and Consistent Expectations:** Establish clear rules and expectations, using simple language and visual aids if needed. Consistency across environments is crucial.
- **Empowerment Through Choice and Support:** Offer choices and break down tasks into manageable steps, fostering a sense of control and promoting positive behavior.
- **Patience and Individuality:** Remember, every child is unique. Be patient, experiment with different approaches, and celebrate even small improvements.

Shaping Behavior Through Positive Strategies

Positive reinforcement techniques encourage desired behaviors.

- **The Power of Redirection:** When challenging behaviors arise, gently guide your child towards a different activity or offer choices to distract them.
- **Positive Reinforcement in Action:** Praise desired behaviors with verbal affirmations, affection, or a reward system. Focus on the positive and tailor the approach to your child's needs.
- **Seeking Professional Guidance:** Do not hesitate to consult therapists or behavior specialists for personalized advice and support in implementing these techniques effectively.

Developing a Consistent Behavior Plan

A collaborative approach with professionals fosters long-term success.

- **Teamwork with Therapists and Educators:** Work with therapists and educators to understand triggers, develop a behavior plan, and implement it consistently across home and school settings.
- **Goal Setting and Shared Values:** Establish clear goals and values for the behavior plan, focusing on positive behavior reinforcement, preventing challenging behaviors, and teaching alternative coping strategies.
- **Celebrating Progress and Seeking Support:** Acknowledge and celebrate your child's progress, no matter how small. Remember, you are not alone. Seek additional support from therapists, advocacy groups, or other professionals if needed.

Positive behavior support techniques are essential tools for helping children with CP manage their behaviors effectively. By understanding triggers, utilizing redirection and positive reinforcement, and collaborating with professionals to develop a consistent plan, you can create a supportive environment where your child thrives, learns appropriate behaviors, and builds confidence to navigate their world successfully.

Building Coping Mechanisms

Cerebral Palsy (CP) can present physical and emotional challenges for children. This section explores the importance of teaching relaxation techniques, promoting emotional regulation skills, and seeking professional help when needed, to equip children with CP with effective coping mechanisms.

Teaching Relaxation Techniques

Relaxation techniques empower children to manage stress and muscle tension.

- **Tailored Techniques:** Choose age-appropriate and engaging techniques, like deep breathing or visualization of calming environments.
- **Gamification and Consistency:** Turn relaxation into a game or integrate it into bedtime routines. Regular practice is key.
- **Modeling and Positive Reinforcement:** Practice relaxation techniques yourself and celebrate your child's efforts, promoting a positive and calming association.
- **Identifying Stressors:** Openly discuss what causes stress and collaboratively develop coping mechanisms to address these triggers.

Promoting Emotional Regulation Skills

Emotional regulation empowers children to manage their feelings effectively.

- **Validation and Emotional Vocabulary:** Acknowledge the validity of all emotions, and help them identify and express their feelings using appropriate vocabulary.

- **Leading by Example:** Model healthy ways to manage your own emotions, providing a positive example for your child.
- **Creating a Safe Space:** Establish a designated quiet space where your child can relax and regulate their emotions when overwhelmed.
- **Positive Reinforcement and Patience:** Celebrate their attempts at emotional regulation, and remember, developing these skills takes time and consistent support.
- **Professional Guidance:** Seek resources from therapists, books, or websites specializing in emotional development for children.

Seeking Professional Help

There is no shame in seeking professional support.
- **Identifying Signs of Difficulty:** Be mindful of indicators your child might need additional support, such as frequent tantrums, social withdrawal, or changes in sleep patterns.
- **Building a Support Team:** Consult your child's doctor for referrals to therapists or counselors specializing in CP. Different types of professionals can offer support, including child therapists, physical therapists, occupational therapists, and speech-language pathologists.
- **Collaboration and Open Communication:** Actively participate in your child's therapy, communicate openly with the therapist, and work collaboratively with other caregivers to ensure consistent support across environments.
- **Strength in Seeking Help:** Remember, seeking professional help demonstrates your commitment to your child's well-being, and therapy can equip them with valuable tools to navigate challenges and thrive.

Building coping mechanisms is essential for children with CP to manage stress, regulate emotions, and navigate life's challenges with confidence. By teaching relaxation techniques, fostering emotional regulation skills, and seeking professional support when needed, you can empower your child to develop resilience and build a brighter future.

Finding Support for Mental Health Concerns

Cerebral Palsy (CP) can present unique mental health challenges for children. This section explores strategies for identifying qualified mental health professionals, the benefits of support groups, and navigating available resources to ensure your child's well-being.

Finding Qualified Mental Health Professionals

Finding the right mental health professional is crucial for effective support.

- **Pediatrician's Guidance:** Start by consulting your child's pediatrician for referrals to therapists or counselors specializing in CP. Their expertise can connect you with qualified professionals.
- **Network and Online Resources:** Utilize your network of family, friends, and healthcare providers for recommendations. Online resources like professional association websites can provide directories of specialists in your area.
- **Considering Practicalities:** Factor in location, insurance coverage, and your child's comfort level when selecting a therapist.
- **Open Communication and Collaboration:** Prepare a list of concerns beforehand and involve your child if possible, during the initial consultation to facilitate open communication and collaboration with the therapist.
- **Strength in Seeking Help:** Remember, seeking professional support demonstrates your commitment to your child's mental health, and can equip them with valuable tools to navigate challenges and thrive.

The Value of Support Groups

Support groups connect you with others facing similar challenges.

- **Finding In-Person or Virtual Groups:** Local hospitals, disability organizations, or mental health providers may offer in-person support groups specifically focused on CP and mental health. Online resources like The Cerebral Palsy Foundation or United Cerebral Palsy can provide virtual support options.
- **Exploring Online Communities:** Consider online communities like Inspire.com or Facebook groups dedicated to CP. These groups can offer valuable peer-to-peer connections and support.
- **Finding the Right Fit:** When choosing a group, consider factors like the focus on mental health, age suitability, format (in-person or virtual), and reach out to the organizer for more information.
- **Managing Stress and Anxiety:** Support groups provide a safe space to share experiences, learn coping mechanisms from others, and reduce feelings of isolation, ultimately aiding in managing stress and anxiety.

Addressing your child's mental health needs is vital for their overall well-being. By leveraging the expertise of qualified professionals, the strength of support groups, and the resources available online and in your community, you can create a comprehensive support system that empowers your child to thrive. Remember, you are not alone on this journey.

8. PROMOTING SOCIAL INCLUSION

Strategies for Building Friendships

Friendship is a cornerstone of social development and well-being. This section explores strategies for helping children with Cerebral Palsy (CP) cultivate meaningful friendships, focusing on encouraging social activity, developing social skills, and fostering empathy and understanding.

Participation in Social Activities and Groups

Creating opportunities for social interaction is crucial.

- **Identifying Interests:** Consider your child's hobbies and interests. Explore activities like adapted sports, art groups, or online gaming communities that cater to their abilities and passions.
- **Accessibility Considerations:** Ensure chosen activities are accessible and inclusive, removing any physical barriers to participation.
- **Supporting Socialization:** Guide your child in initiating interactions and offer strategies like using visuals or role-playing for better communication.
- **Positive Reinforcement and Patience:** Acknowledge and celebrate your child's social efforts. Building friendships takes time, so maintain patience and provide ongoing support.
- **Exploring Support Programs:** Research programs offered by disability organizations or therapists specifically designed to enhance social skills development.

Social Skills Through Play and Communication Programs

Learning social skills paves the way for strong friendships.

- **The Power of Play:** Encourage social interactions through playdates, games with peers, and collaborative activities like art projects. Play fosters communication and relationship building.
- **Communication Therapy:** Speech therapy programs can equip your child with enhanced communication skills, improving their ability to express themselves and understand others.
- **Positive Reinforcement and Support:** Acknowledge your child's efforts to socialize, even if they seem small. Celebrate their progress and offer support as they navigate social interactions.
- **Professional Support Systems:** If you have concerns about your child's social skills, seek guidance from therapists or other professionals who can offer tailored strategies.

Teaching Empathy and Understanding of Differences

Understanding others is key to building strong bonds

- **Open Communication and Celebrating Differences:** Discuss the concept of differences in a positive light, emphasizing your child's unique strengths and celebrating diversity.
- **Promoting Inclusivity:** Encourage your child to play with a variety of peers and participate in volunteer activities that foster empathy and understanding of others' needs.
- **The Power of Media:** Utilize books and shows that portray characters with diverse backgrounds and abilities to promote inclusivity and empathy.
- **Modeling Kindness and Anti-Bullying:** Lead by example, demonstrating kindness and respect towards everyone. Equip your child with strategies to address bullying behavior.
- **Fostering Compassionate Interactions:** By encouraging positive social interactions and celebrating empathy, you help your child build strong and meaningful friendships.

Building friendships enriches a child's life, and children with CP are no exception. Through participation in social activities, development of social skills, and fostering empathy and understanding, you can empower your child to connect with others, form lasting friendships, and experience the joy of belonging.

Remember, your unwavering support and a collaborative approach create the foundation for a fulfilling social life for your child.

Creating Inclusive Playgrounds and Activities

Play is essential for a child's development, fostering physical activity, social skills, and imagination.

This section explores the importance of advocating for accessible playgrounds, finding adapted activities, and promoting inclusive play dates and community events, ensuring all children, including those with Cerebral Palsy (CP), have the right to play.

Building Accessible Playgrounds

Accessibility is key to dismantling barriers to play.

- **Understanding Accessibility Standards:** Educate yourself about playground accessibility regulations. Resources like the Americans with Disabilities Act (ADA) provide guidelines for inclusive play areas.
- **Collaboration and Advocacy:** Connect with other parents and disability organizations to amplify your voice. Work together to advocate for accessible features like ramps, adaptive swings, and sensory-friendly spaces in playgrounds.
- **Raising Awareness:** Speak at community meetings, contact local media, and utilize social media to raise awareness about the importance of inclusive playgrounds. By working together, we can create playgrounds where all children can play side-by-side.

Finding Adapted Activities and Games

Inclusive play goes beyond physical accessibility.

- **Adapting Traditional Games:** Explore creative ways to modify popular games so everyone can participate. Consider walking tag instead of running, or creating tactile sensory bins with different textures.
- **Resource Exploration:** Seek inspiration online or consult therapists for ideas on adapted activities and games that promote engagement for all children.
- **Collaboration for Change:** Discuss ideas with local park authorities regarding inclusive design elements in playgrounds. Spread the word in your community to garner support for creating inclusive play spaces.

Promoting Inclusive Play Dates and Community Events

Social interactions are nurtured through inclusive play.

- **Understanding Your Child's Interests:** Discuss their hobbies and preferences. Connect with other parents who share your desire for inclusive experiences.
- **Planning Activities for All:** Organize play dates or outings with activities everyone can enjoy, considering accessibility and varying abilities.
- **Advocacy for Inclusive Events:** Talk to event organizers about making community events more inclusive. Promote awareness in your neighborhood about the importance of accessibility.
- **Leading by Example:** Demonstrate kindness and acceptance of differences. Celebrate the unique strengths of each child.
- **Finding Support Networks:** Utilize resources from disability organizations and online communities to connect with others who share your vision of inclusion. Together, we can create a

welcoming environment where all children feel valued and empowered to play.

Play is a right, not a privilege. By advocating for accessible playgrounds, finding adapted activities, and promoting inclusive play experiences, we can dismantle barriers and create a world where all children, including those with CP, can play, learn, and build meaningful friendships. Through collaboration, a commitment to inclusion, and a celebration of differences, we can turn playgrounds into spaces of joy and connection for every child.

Addressing Bullying and Social Isolation

Children with Cerebral Palsy (CP) face unique challenges, and bullying can be a devastating experience.

This section explores the importance of recognizing signs of bullying and social exclusion, teaching strategies to respond, and building a support system to empower your child.

Recognizing the Warning Signs

Early intervention is crucial for addressing bullying.

- **Behavioral Changes:** Be vigilant for changes in your child's behavior, such as withdrawal, anxiety, or unexplained injuries.
- **Social Cues:** Pay attention to social cues like sadness after school or difficulty making friends.
- **Open Communication:** Create a safe space for open communication and actively listen to your child's concerns. Discuss bullying openly and build their confidence.
- **Documentation and Support:** If bullying is suspected, document incidents, talk to teachers and counselors, and consider

seeking support from other parents. Your vigilance can ensure your child feels safe and valued at school.

Teaching Strategies to Address Bullying

Equipping your child with coping mechanisms is essential.

- **Building Confidence:** Focus on your child's strengths and encourage positive self-talk. A strong sense of self empowers them to navigate challenges.
- **Developing Coping Strategies:** Teach them to stay calm, walk away from bullies, and seek help from trusted adults. Practice different bullying scenarios together.
- **Assertiveness and Support Networks:** Discuss cyberbullying and assertive communication. Highlight the importance of helping others who are bullied and building strong support networks. With your guidance, your child can learn to stand up for themselves and feel confident.

Support Systems and Reporting Incidents

A collaborative approach is key to combating bullying.

- **Building a Support Network:** Create a strong support system with family, friends, therapists, and disability organizations. Having a network of advocates empowers you and your child.
- **Open Communication and Documentation:** Maintain open communication with your child about bullying. Document any incidents thoroughly.
- **Reporting and Advocacy:** Report bullying to the school and understand your rights under anti-bullying laws. Seek support from advocacy groups if needed. Remember, you are not alone.

Bullying can be a painful experience, but with awareness, intervention, and a strong support system, you can empower your child to navigate social challenges and build resilience. By recognizing the signs of bullying, teaching effective coping strategies, and collaborating with others, you can create a safe and inclusive environment where your child with CP can thrive and reach their full potential.

The Importance of Peer Support & Role Models

Social connection and positive role models are essential for a child's development.

This section explores the significance of encouraging interaction with typically developing peers, identifying positive role models with CP, and the benefits of peer mentorship programs for children with Cerebral Palsy (CP).

Encouraging Interaction with Typically Developing Peers

Peer interaction fosters social and emotional growth.

- **Creating Inclusive Opportunities:** Involve your child in activities with typically developing peers, such as school clubs, community events, or playdates.
- **Promoting Strengths and Patience:** Prepare your child by highlighting their strengths and offering positive reinforcement. Social interaction takes time and practice, so be patient and supportive.
- **Advocacy and Education:** Advocate for inclusive spaces and educate others about CP to create a welcoming and understanding environment.
- **Friendship and Growth:** By fostering these interactions, you empower your child to build friendships, develop social skills, and gain confidence.

Identifying Positive Role Models with CP

Role models offer a vision of possibilities.

- **Seeking Diverse Inspiration:** Search for positive role models with CP across different ages, interests, and achievements. Disability organizations, online communities, and media can be valuable resources.
- **Connecting with Role Models:** Encourage your child to follow their role models online, watch interviews, or write letters, fostering a sense of connection.
- **Empowerment and Self-Belief:** Seeing others with CP achieve their goals can inspire your child to set ambitious goals, believe in themselves, and develop self-advocacy skills.
- **Acceptance and Reduced Stigma:** Role models normalize CP and promote acceptance within society. They empower your child to embrace their unique journey.

The Benefits of Peer Mentorship Programs

Peer mentors provide friendship and guidance.

- **Finding the Right Fit:** Seek peer mentorship programs that match your child's age, interests, and needs. Mentors can be older students or young adults without disabilities.
- **Social Skills Development and Confidence:** Through interaction with mentors, your child can develop social skills, gain confidence, and find a positive role model close in age.
- **Open Communication and Positive Experiences:** Maintain open communication with your child and the program coordinator to ensure a positive and enriching experience.
- **Building Friendships and Social Success:** Peer mentorship programs provide opportunities for building friendships, fostering social inclusion, and empowering your child to thrive.

Peer support and role models offer invaluable guidance and inspiration for children with CP. By encouraging interaction with typically developing peers, identifying positive role models, and exploring peer mentorship programs, you can create a rich social tapestry that empowers your child to build meaningful connections, develop essential social skills, and navigate their world with confidence.

Remember, fostering a supportive network is key to unlocking your child's full potential.

Building Self-Advocacy Skills

Self-advocacy empowers individuals to communicate their needs, wants, and desires effectively.

This section explores strategies for teaching children with Cerebral Palsy (CP) to build strong self-advocacy skills, fostering confidence and independence.

Communication and Choice

Effective communication is the cornerstone of self-advocacy.

- **Early Intervention:** Begin fostering self-advocacy skills early. Provide choices, even small ones, and celebrate their attempts to communicate their preferences.
- **Finding the Right Voice:** Help your child discover the most effective way for them to express themselves, utilizing pictures, assistive technology, or sign language if necessary.
- **Building Independence:** Gradually increase opportunities for your child to make choices, fostering a sense of autonomy and decision-making skills.

Role-Playing and Reinforcement

Repetition and positive reinforcement solidify self-advocacy.

- **Safe Space for Practice:** Create a safe and supportive environment for role-playing scenarios where your child can practice expressing their needs.
- **Positive Reinforcement:** Acknowledge and celebrate their attempts at self-advocacy, no matter how small. Positive reinforcement builds confidence.
- **Embracing Communication Styles:** Be open to and supportive of different communication styles your child may develop.

Working with Professionals

Collaboration strengthens the foundation of self-advocacy.

- **Teamwork with Therapists and Educators:** Work with therapists, teachers, and caregivers to ensure consistent practice and reinforcement of self-advocacy skills across different environments.
- **Building Self-Esteem:** Highlight your child's strengths and accomplishments, fostering a strong sense of self-worth and confidence. This empowers them to communicate effectively.

Building Self-Belief and Assertiveness

Confidence is key to effective self-advocacy.

- **Celebrating Achievements:** Celebrate your child's successes and achievements, big or small. Focus on progress and their unique strengths.

- **Decision-Making and Problem-Solving:** Encourage them to make decisions by offering age-appropriate choices and respecting their opinions. Problem-solving together builds confidence.
- **Social Interaction and Role Models:** Support positive social interactions with peers and foster healthy relationships. Expose them to role models with CP who excel in various fields.
- **Focusing on Abilities:** Shift the focus from limitations to abilities. This empowers your child to face challenges with confidence and advocate for themselves.

Self-advocacy empowers children with CP to navigate life with confidence and independence. By nurturing early communication skills, providing opportunities for choice, offering positive reinforcement for self-advocacy attempts, and fostering a strong sense of self-worth, you can equip your child with the tools they need to find their voice and thrive in the world.

Remember, your unwavering support is key to their success.

Providing Opportunities for Practice in Different Settings

Self-advocacy empowers individuals to express their needs and navigate life independently.

This section explores the importance of providing children with Cerebral Palsy (CP) with opportunities to practice self-advocacy skills in various settings, fostering confidence and a strong voice.

A Safe Space for Exploration

The home environment provides a foundation for self-advocacy.

- **Empowering Choices:** Start by offering choices, even small ones, at home. Encourage them to communicate their needs and preferences.
- **Role-Playing for Real-Life:** Practice everyday scenarios through role-playing, like ordering food, requesting help, or expressing discomfort. This equips them for real-world situations.

Stepping Out into the Community

As your child develops, expand practice opportunities.

- **Doctor's Appointments:** Involve your child in doctor's visits, encouraging them to answer questions and express concerns where possible.
- **School Activities:** Promote self-advocacy in school by supporting their participation in activities, allowing them to speak up for themselves in class discussions or with teachers.

Everyday Moments of Teachable Opportunities

Daily interactions offer valuable lessons.

- **Turning Everyday Moments into Learning Experiences:** Use everyday situations to discuss self-advocacy and its importance. Help them understand how to express their needs effectively.
- **Positive Reinforcement and Patience:** Celebrate their efforts at self-advocacy, no matter how small. Be patient as they develop their voice and confidence over time.

Self-advocacy is a journey, not a destination. By providing opportunities for practice in a safe and supportive home environment, gradually expanding these opportunities into the community and schools, and celebrating every step along the way, you can empower your child with CP to develop the confidence and skills they need to navigate life with independence and self-assurance. Remember, your unwavering support is key to their success in building a strong voice and advocating for themselves.

9. HEALTH & WELLNESS THROUGHOUT LIFE

Maintaining a Healthy Lifestyle

Cerebral Palsy (CP) presents unique challenges, but promoting a healthy lifestyle empowers children with CP to thrive.

This section explores key aspects of maintaining a healthy lifestyle, focusing on a balanced diet, regular physical activity, and the importance of preventive healthcare.

A Balanced Dietary Approach

Nutrition plays a pivotal role in a child's overall health.

- **Building a Balanced Plate:** Prioritize a diet rich in fruits, vegetables, whole grains, lean proteins, and healthy fats. These provide essential nutrients for growth and development.
- **Calcium for Strong Bones:** Incorporate dairy products for a healthy dose of calcium, crucial for strong bone health.
- **Hydration is Key:** Ensure adequate hydration by encouraging frequent water intake.
- **Modified Textures and Speech Therapy:** If chewing or swallowing presents difficulties, adjust food textures as needed. Consult a speech therapist to address swallowing concerns and develop safe eating strategies.
- **Calorie Requirements:** Increased muscle activity in children with CP can necessitate higher calorie intake. Discuss portion sizes with your pediatrician to ensure proper growth.
- **Engaging Mealtimes:** Involve your child in meal planning and make mealtimes fun. This fosters healthy eating habits and a positive relationship with food.

Promoting Activity and Well-being

Regular physical activity offers numerous benefits.

- **Consulting Healthcare Professionals:** Collaborate with your child's doctor and therapist to design safe and appropriate exercise programs.
- **Tailored Activities:** Prioritize activities your child enjoys, such as adapted sports or playful exercises, to promote engagement.
- **Identifying Resources:** Explore resources for adapted exercise programs offered by physical therapy practices, community sports programs, or online platforms.
- **Gradual Progression:** Begin exercise programs slowly and gradually increase intensity to avoid overexertion.
- **Celebrating Progress:** Maintain a positive and encouraging environment. Celebrate your child's achievements and milestones to keep them motivated.

Safeguarding Oral and Visual Health

Prioritizing preventive healthcare ensures well-being.

- **Dental Care Considerations:** Children with CP may face unique dental challenges. Start dental visits early, desensitize them to the environment, and utilize adaptive brushing techniques. Limit sugary foods and drinks to maintain good oral hygiene.
- **Vision Care Strategies:** Schedule regular eye exams and communicate effectively with your child's ophthalmologist about their vision. Explore adaptive technology to enhance visual experience.
- **Collaboration with Therapists:** Work with therapists to develop motor skills that improve oral hygiene practices.
- **Celebrating Efforts:** Acknowledge and celebrate your child's efforts in maintaining good oral and visual health.

By prioritizing a balanced diet, engaging in regular physical activity, and maintaining a focus on preventive healthcare, you can contribute significantly to your child's well-being.

Remember, a healthy lifestyle empowers children with CP to reach their full potential and experience a fulfilling life.

Managing Chronic Conditions

Cerebral Palsy (CP) presents a unique set of chronic conditions that require ongoing management.

This section explores strategies for managing pain, addressing fatigue, and monitoring respiratory issues to optimize a child's well-being.

Pain Management Strategies

Pain management is crucial for a child's comfort and quality of life.

- **Identifying Pain Signals:** Be attentive to changes in behavior, sleep patterns, or facial expressions that might indicate pain. Open communication with your child is essential.
- **Identifying the Source:** Collaborate with your child's doctor to pinpoint the cause of pain, such as muscle stiffness, medication side effects, or other factors.
- **Non-Medication Approaches:** Prioritize non-medication strategies like physical therapy, heat or cold therapy, massage, and assistive devices to manage pain.
- **Medication Considerations:** If necessary, follow your doctor's instructions carefully when using prescription medications for pain control.
- **Pain Diary and Support:** Maintain a pain diary to track episodes. Create a calm environment during flare-ups and provide ongoing support with daily activities.

Combating Fatigue

Fatigue can be a significant hurdle for children with CP.

- **Understanding the Cause:** Identify underlying factors contributing to fatigue, such as muscle exertion, pain, sleep issues, or nutritional deficiencies.
- **Promoting Activity and Energy Conservation:** Encourage regular physical activity tailored to your child's abilities, such as swimming or yoga. Teach them energy conservation techniques to optimize their endurance.
- **Holistic Approach:** Collaborate with healthcare professionals to manage pain effectively and establish a consistent sleep routine. Ensure a balanced diet, adequate hydration, and explore medication if needed.
- **Monitoring Energy Levels and Support:** Monitor your child's energy levels, schedule breaks throughout the day, and provide positive reinforcement for their efforts. Maintain open communication and seek support from healthcare professionals and disability organizations.

Ensuring Respiratory Health

Muscle control issues in children with CP can affect their breathing.

- **Identifying Signs of Respiratory Distress:** Be vigilant for signs like rapid breathing, wheezing, coughing, or changes in chest movement. Track and report any concerning symptoms to your doctor.
- **Positioning and Physical Therapy:** Proper positioning can improve lung function. Consider chest physical therapy if recommended by your doctor.
- **Vaccinations and Preventive Care:** Keep your child's vaccinations up-to-date to minimize respiratory illnesses. Minimize

exposure to smoke and promote a healthy lifestyle with a balanced diet and regular exercise.

- **Early Intervention and Proactive Management:** Seek immediate medical attention for any breathing problems. By staying alert and taking proactive steps, you can contribute to your child's lung health and overall well-being.

Managing chronic conditions in children with CP requires a multi-faceted approach. By implementing effective pain management strategies, addressing fatigue, and proactively monitoring respiratory health, you can empower your child to thrive despite these challenges.

Remember, collaboration with healthcare professionals, open communication with your child, and unwavering support are key to navigating these challenges and ensuring your child's quality of life.

Transitioning to Adult Healthcare Systems

The journey of a child with Cerebral Palsy (CP) extends beyond pediatrics. This section explores key considerations for a successful transition to adult healthcare, focusing on finding qualified providers, understanding adult medical care, and fostering patient autonomy.

Finding Adult Healthcare Professionals with CP Expertise

Early planning is crucial for a smooth transition.

- **Initiating the Conversation:** Begin discussions with your child's pediatrician as early as age 14-16 to establish a timeline and identify potential challenges.
- **Identifying Qualified Providers:** Research adult healthcare professionals with experience treating CP. Utilize resources like specialty clinics, CP organizations, online directories, and

recommendations from other parents. Prioritize factors like CP expertise, clear communication skills, and accessibility.

- **Medical Records and Continuity of Care:** Gather comprehensive medical records for a seamless transfer of information to the new healthcare provider. Schedule a joint appointment with both the pediatrician and adult healthcare professional to facilitate a smooth transition.

- **Preparing Your Child and Advocating for Their Needs:** Prepare your child for the changes and empower them to be active participants in their healthcare. Be their advocate during appointments, ensuring their questions and concerns are addressed.

- **Multidisciplinary Care:** Consider the potential need for a multidisciplinary team of specialists for comprehensive care. Explore support services offered by adult healthcare facilities to optimize your child's well-being.

Understanding Adult Medical Care Procedures

Knowledge empowers informed decision-making.

- **Understanding the System:** Recognize the differences between pediatric and adult healthcare. Learn about insurance regulations, appointment scheduling, referral processes, and patient billing.

- **Finding CP-Experienced Providers:** Seek adult healthcare professionals specifically experienced in treating CP. This ensures a deeper understanding of your child's needs and potential complications.

- **Medical Knowledge and Communication:** Gain a basic understanding of medical terminology relevant to CP and your child's specific conditions. Develop a communication plan with your child to facilitate effective communication during appointments.

- **Empowering Your Child:** Practice advocating for their needs during appointments. Encourage them to ask questions and express concerns openly.
- **Joint Appointments and Support Resources:** Schedule a joint appointment with your child's pediatrician and new adult doctor to bridge the gap between healthcare systems. Utilize resources offered by organizations like The Cerebral Palsy Foundation, United Cerebral Palsy, NIH, and disability rights organizations for guidance and support.

Patient Autonomy and Shared Decision-Making

Transitioning to adult healthcare is an opportunity to empower your child.

- **Supporting Patient Autonomy:** Respect your child's right to make healthcare decisions. Encourage them to participate in discussions and co-create treatment plans with healthcare professionals.
- **Involving Your Child Early On:** Gradually involve your child in healthcare discussions as they mature. Respect their opinions and preferences.
- **Building Responsibility:** Encourage your child to take on more responsibility for their healthcare routine as they age. This includes self-management of medications, appointment scheduling, and communication with healthcare providers.
- **Shared Decision-Making:** Open communication is key. Gather information together, discuss treatment options, and empower your child to participate actively in decision-making.
- **Preparation and Teamwork:** Prepare for adult healthcare by researching specialists, practicing communication strategies, and ensuring a smooth transfer of medical records. Remember, you are a team working together to support your child's transition and future health.

Transitioning to adult healthcare can feel overwhelming for children with CP and their families. However, by planning ahead, finding qualified professionals, understanding adult healthcare procedures, and fostering patient autonomy, you can empower your child to navigate this transition with confidence and take charge of their well-being.

Remember, support and collaboration are key ingredients for a successful journey into adulthood.

Importance of Regular Medical Checkups

Cerebral Palsy (CP) presents unique medical needs, making regular checkups even more crucial for children with this condition.

This section explores the significance of preventive care appointments, monitoring growth and development, and early detection of potential health concerns.

Scheduling Preventive Care Appointments

Preventive care is the cornerstone of maintaining a child's health.

- **Establishing a Schedule:** Collaborate with your child's doctor to establish a preventive care schedule tailored to their age and specific medical needs. This may include regular physicals, vaccinations, and specialist consultations, if necessary.
- **Accessibility and Comfort:** Consider factors like appointment times, location accessibility, and your child's comfort level when scheduling appointments.
- **Preparation and Advocacy:** Prepare for each appointment by gathering relevant information, such as medication lists and recent health concerns. Advocate for your child's needs and ensure clear communication with the healthcare team.

- **Resources and Optimization:** Utilize resources from organizations like the CDC and AAP to create an effective vaccination and screening plan. By prioritizing preventive care, you contribute significantly to your child's well-being and empower them to thrive.

Monitoring Development Throughout Life

Closely monitoring growth and development is essential for children with CP.

- **Comprehensive Checkups:** Regular checkups with the doctor provide an opportunity to monitor physical growth, track developmental milestones, and address any medical issues.
- **Proactive Management:** These appointments are vital for ensuring children with CP receive necessary vaccinations and screenings for potential complications.
- **Observational Support at Home:** Supplement doctor visits by observing your child's progress at home, tracking milestones, and maintaining a doctor-provided growth chart.
- **Open Communication and Celebration:** Maintain open communication with the healthcare team regarding your observations. Celebrate your child's achievements, big or small, to foster confidence in their abilities.

Early Detection of Potential Health Concerns

Regular checkups are critical for early detection of potential health concerns.

- **Proactive Detection:** Early detection allows for prompt intervention and treatment before symptoms worsen. This can significantly improve outcomes and overall well-being.

- **Open Communication and Observation:** Be open with the doctor about any changes in your child's movement, behavior, pain levels, or sleep patterns.
- **Comprehensive Assessment:** Discuss with the doctor your child's development, vision, hearing, nutrition, and emotional well-being.
- **Advocacy and Information Gathering:** Maintain a journal of your child's health to track trends and prepare a list of questions for each appointment. Advocate for your child's needs and ensure all concerns are addressed.

Regular medical checkups are a cornerstone of optimal health for children with CP. By prioritizing preventive care, monitoring growth and development, and facilitating early detection of health concerns, you empower your child to thrive and live a fulfilling life. Remember, a strong partnership with your child's healthcare team and unwavering support are crucial for navigating this journey together.

Sexuality and Relationship Education

Sexuality and relationships are fundamental aspects of human experience.

This section explores the importance of providing children with Cerebral Palsy (CP) with age-appropriate education, promoting healthy body image and self-esteem, and addressing their specific needs and concerns.

Providing Age-Appropriate Education

Open communication empowers informed decision-making.

- **Tailored Approach:** Begin with simple concepts like body parts and hygiene when children are young. Gradually introduce more complex topics like puberty and consent as they mature.
- **Clear Communication and Openness:** Use clear, non-judgmental language and encourage them to ask questions freely.
- **Resource Utilization:** Consider seeking support from therapists, disability organizations, or websites which offer resources specifically for sexuality education.
- **Building Confidence and Trust:** By having open conversations, you empower your child to navigate relationships with confidence and self-respect.

Promoting Healthy Body Image and Self-Esteem

Supporting a positive self-image is crucial for well-being.

- **Positive Body Image Role Modeling:** Lead by example and promote a positive body image for yourself.
- **Celebrating Strengths and Accomplishments:** Shift the focus to your child's unique talents and achievements, fostering self-worth.
- **Celebrating Differences:** Challenge societal stereotypes and expose your child to positive representations of people with disabilities.
- **Healthy Habits and Inner Beauty:** Encourage healthy lifestyle choices like good nutrition and physical activity. Reinforce the message that inner beauty and health are more important than appearance.
- **Celebrating Uniqueness:** Highlight your child's unique personality and talents, fostering self-acceptance.
- **Open Communication and Support:** Maintain open communication channels so your child feels comfortable expressing their feelings. Seek professional support from therapists if needed.

Addressing Individual Needs

Adapting communication strategies is essential for effective dialogue.

- **Age-Appropriate Communication:** Tailor communication to your child's age and developmental level. Use simple language and focus on feelings for younger children.
- **Creating a Safe Space:** Assure your child they can talk to you about anything without judgment. Listen actively and encourage open communication.
- **Exploring Emotions and Challenges:** Discuss their feelings openly, validating their experiences. Talk about challenges related to CP and brainstorm solutions together.
- **Healthy Coping Mechanisms:** Equip your child with healthy ways to manage stress or social anxieties.
- **Celebrating Achievements:** Recognize and celebrate all achievements, big or small, to reinforce their self-confidence.
- **Professional Support:** Consider seeking professional support from therapists trained in communication strategies for children with CP.

Sexuality and relationship education, a positive body image, and open communication are fundamental building blocks for a child with CP to develop healthy relationships and navigate life with confidence. By providing age-appropriate education, fostering self-esteem, and addressing their specific needs, you empower your child to embrace their individuality and thrive.

Remember, open communication, unwavering support, and a collaborative approach are key to navigating this journey together.

10. FINANCIAL PLANNING & BENEFITS

Understanding Government Programs & Benefits

Raising a child with Cerebral Palsy (CP) presents unique challenges, including potential financial burdens.

This section explores the process of qualifying for Social Security Disability Insurance (SSDI) for your child, highlighting key considerations and available resources.

Eligibility Requirements

The Social Security Administration (SSA) offers two primary programs.

- **Supplemental Security Income (SSI):** This program provides financial support for individuals with limited income and resources, regardless of work history. However, it may not be readily available for children with working parents.
- **Social Security Disability Insurance (SSDI):** This program offers benefits to children whose parents have a sufficient work history and paid Social Security taxes. SSDI eligibility hinges on the severity of your child's CP.

Criteria for SSDI Qualification

- **Functional Limitations:** Your child's CP must significantly impact their ability to perform daily activities such as walking, dressing, or attending school.
- **Medical Documentation:** Strong medical evidence from specialists documenting your child's condition and limitations is crucial for a successful application.

The Application Process

- **Online or In-Person:** Applications can be submitted online or through your local SSA office.
- **Denied Applications and Appeals:** Initial applications are often denied. However, you have the right to appeal with the support of an attorney specializing in disability law.

Available Resources

- **Social Security Administration Website:** The SSA website provides comprehensive information on the application process, eligibility requirements, and valuable resources.
- **Cerebral Palsy Foundation:** Organizations like the Cerebral Palsy Foundation offer guidance and support throughout the application process.

Key Considerations

- **Patience and Persistence:** The SSDI application process can be lengthy. Be patient, gather strong documentation, and seek professional help if needed.
- **Advocating for Your Child:** Be your child's advocate by presenting a clear picture of their limitations and the impact of CP on their daily life.

Securing SSDI benefits can significantly ease the financial burden of raising a child with CP. By understanding the criteria, gathering strong documentation, and utilizing available resources, you can increase your chances of a successful application.

Remember, advocating for your child and seeking support can help ensure they receive the financial assistance they deserve.

Health Insurance Considerations & Advocacy

Cerebral Palsy (CP) presents a unique set of challenges, and navigating the complexities of health insurance to secure necessary treatment is paramount.

This section explores understanding insurance coverage for CP treatment, appealing denials, and finding resources for advocacy.

Key Considerations for CP Treatment

A clear understanding of your insurance plan is vital.

- **Covered Services:** Most plans cover essential therapies like physical, occupational, and speech therapy, assistive technology, and medications for managing CP symptoms.
- **Plan Specificity:** Review your specific plan details to identify covered services and potential exclusions.
- **Pre-Authorization:** Certain treatments might require pre-authorization from your insurance provider. Discuss this with your child's doctor to ensure smooth treatment initiation.

Managing Costs and Utilizing Resources

- **In-Network Providers:** Utilizing in-network providers typically translates to lower costs.
- **Understanding Costs:** Familiarize yourself with terms like deductibles, copayments, and out-of-pocket maximums to effectively manage out-of-pocket expenses.
- **Record Keeping:** Maintain meticulous records of medical bills and insurance paperwork for future reference.
- **Seeking Support:** Do not hesitate to seek guidance from your child's doctor or organizations specializing in CP care and advocacy.

Appealing Denials

Insurance denials should not deter you from securing necessary treatment.

- **Understanding the Denial:** The Explanation of Review (EOR) from your insurance company explains the rationale behind the denial. Review it thoroughly.
- **Gathering Evidence:** Collect all medical records demonstrating the necessity of the denied treatment.
- **The Appeal Process:** Contact your insurance company to initiate the appeal process. Write a clear and concise appeal letter outlining the medical justification for the treatment and include supporting documents.
- **Independent Review:** If necessary, request an independent medical review for impartial evaluation.
- **Requesting a Hearing:** In case of a second denial, consider requesting a hearing and prepare diligently for it.

Advocacy and Support

Numerous resources exist to aid you in navigating insurance complexities.

- **Disability Organizations:** Organizations like the Cerebral Palsy Foundation and United Cerebral Palsy offer valuable resources and guidance on insurance matters.
- **Hospital Social Workers:** Social workers at hospitals can provide support and assistance with insurance challenges.
- **Legal Aid:** If needed, legal aid organizations can offer legal representation during appeals.
- **Staying Informed:** Maintain a proactive approach by staying informed about relevant laws and regulations.

The journey of raising a child with CP is demanding, but you are not alone. By understanding your insurance plan, persistently advocating for coverage through appeals, and utilizing available support systems, you can ensure your child receives the vital treatment they deserve.

Remember, your unwavering advocacy empowers you to navigate the complexities of healthcare insurance and secure the best possible care for your child.

Educational Funding & Scholarships

The pursuit of higher education should be accessible to all, but for students with Cerebral Palsy (CP), the financial burden can seem insurmountable. This section explores strategies for navigating this challenge, focusing on exploring financial aid options, identifying scholarships and grants, and advocating for inclusive educational opportunities.

Financial Aid Resources

Multiple avenues exist to ease the financial burden of college.

- **Federal Grants and Loans:** Explore federal financial aid options like Grants and Direct Subsidized Loans. These programs offer need-based financial assistance that can significantly reduce tuition costs.
- **State Grants and Scholarships:** Contact your state's Department of Education to discover state-specific grants and scholarships. These programs often cater to students with disabilities, offering additional support.
- **Institutional Aid:** Many colleges and universities offer financial aid specifically for students with disabilities. Reach out to their financial aid offices to learn more about available programs.

Optimizing the Funding through Early Planning

Planning and proactive measures are crucial for maximizing financial aid opportunities.

- **Filing the FAFSA:** The Free Application for Federal Student Aid (FAFSA) is the gateway to federal and state financial aid. Start early each year to ensure timely processing.
- **Dedicated Scholarship Search:** Devote time to researching scholarships. Consider disability-focused resources offered by organizations like the Cerebral Palsy Foundation or United Cerebral Palsy.
- **Financial Aid Office Support:** Do not hesitate to seek help from financial aid offices. They are valuable resources for navigating the application process and identifying additional aid opportunities.

Navigating the Scholarship Landscape

Finding scholarships requires a strategic approach.

- **Local Resources:** Begin your search by checking with your child's school or local organizations that might offer scholarship programs for students with CP.
- **National Resources:** Expand your search to national resources such as government websites and disability organizations dedicated to CP. These resources often compile comprehensive lists of scholarship opportunities.
- **Scholarship Search Engines:** Utilize online scholarship search engines to identify relevant opportunities. Consider disability-focused search engines to refine your results.
- **Professional Associations and Foundations:** Explore scholarship programs offered by professional associations and foundations related to your child's field of study.

- **Early Application and Multiple Opportunities:** Start searching for scholarships as early as possible. Carefully read application requirements, highlight your child's academic achievements and experiences, and apply for multiple scholarships to increase your chances of success.
- **Seeking Help:** Do not hesitate to seek assistance from organizations specializing in scholarships for students with disabilities.

Inclusion for Educational Opportunities

Every child deserves access to quality education.

- **Understanding Your Rights:** Familiarize yourself with laws like the Individuals with Disabilities Education Act (IDEA), which guarantees a free and appropriate public education (FAPE) for students with disabilities.
- **Understanding CP:** Gain a comprehensive understanding of CP and its potential impact on learning.
- **Gathering Information:** Collaborate with doctors, therapists, and teachers to create a detailed picture of your child's specific needs.
- **Open Communication with Schools:** Maintain regular communication with teachers and school staff. Share information about your child and advocate for the support they require to succeed.
- **Positive and Proactive Approach:** Maintain a positive and respectful approach during interactions with educators. Ask questions and collaborate to create a learning environment that fosters your child's academic and personal growth.
- **Support Organizations and Empowering Your Child:** Utilize resources offered by organizations specializing in disability advocacy. As your child matures, include them in discussions and decisions regarding their education.

The road to higher education for students with CP requires dedication, creative financing strategies, and unwavering advocacy. By exploring financial aid options, identifying scholarships, and championing inclusive educational opportunities, you can empower your child to achieve their academic dreams and reach their full potential.

Remember, you are not alone in this journey. There are numerous resources available to ensure your child receives the education and support they deserve.

Planning for Long-Term Care Needs

Cerebral Palsy (CP) presents a unique path for individuals and their families. This section explores key considerations for long-term care planning, focusing on future living arrangements, exploring financial tools, and involving your child in the decision-making process.

Envisioning Living Arrangements

As your child with CP matures, considering their future living environment is crucial.

- **Understanding Needs:** Evaluate your child's current level of independence in daily activities, mobility, and medical requirements.
- **Living Options:** Explore a range of possibilities, including independent living with accessibility features, supported living arrangements with daily assistance, group homes offering 24/7 care, or remaining at home with family support.
- **Support Services:** Consider options like personal care assistants, home healthcare services, or vocational rehabilitation programs to help with employment.

Planning for Financial Security

Financial security is essential for long-term care.

- **Cost Estimation:** Begin by estimating your child's current and future expenses, including therapy, potential living costs, and assistive technology needs.
- **Government Benefits:** Explore available government programs like Social Security Disability Insurance (SSDI) to supplement your financial resources.
- **Financial Strategies:** Utilize financial tools like Special Needs Trusts to manage assets while preserving eligibility for government benefits. Consider Health Savings Accounts (HSAs) to set aside funds for qualified medical expenses.
- **Seeking Guidance:** Consult with financial advisors and attorneys specializing in disability planning to create a personalized financial strategy for your child's future.

Shared Decision-Making

Involving your child in planning discussions empowers them and fosters a sense of control.

- **Age-Appropriate Communication:** Tailor your approach based on your child's age. For younger children, use simple choices, pictures, and role-playing.
- **Open Communication and Respect:** As your child matures, engage in open discussions, brainstorm ideas, and acknowledge their thoughts even if they differ from yours.
- **Shifting Focus:** Focus on your child's abilities and encourage them to explore options for education, work, or independent living.
- **Building Confidence and Celebrating Successes:** Create a safe space for open communication and celebrate their successes,

big and small. Seek professional support if needed to facilitate these discussions.

Long-term care planning for a child with CP is a journey of love, responsibility, and proactive planning. By considering living arrangements, exploring financial tools, and involving your child in planning discussions, you can contribute to building a secure and fulfilling future for them. Remember, you are not alone. Numerous resources and support systems are available to guide you along the way.

Estate Planning & Financial Security

Raising a child with Cerebral Palsy (CP) is a journey filled with love and unique challenges.

This section explores the importance of estate planning and financial security for your child's future, focusing on creating a will and special needs trusts, ensuring long-term financial stability, and seeking professional guidance.

Wills and Guardianship

A well-crafted estate plan provides peace of mind.

- **The Legal Document:** A will is a legal document outlining the distribution of your assets upon passing. It can also designate a guardian for your child with CP.
- **Choosing the Guardian:** Select a responsible individual who knows and loves your child well. Discuss your child's needs and wishes with them to ensure continuity of care.
- **Professional Guidance:** Consider consulting an attorney specializing in special needs to navigate the legal complexities and ensure your child's future is protected.

- **Adaptability and Review:** Remember, your estate plan should be a living document. Review and update it as circumstances change.

Building a Financial Safety Net

Proactive financial planning ensures your child's well-being.

- **Government Benefits:** Explore government programs like Social Security Disability Insurance (SSDI) or Supplemental Security Income (SSI) to supplement your income and potentially provide benefits for your child.
- **Cost Estimation and Financial Tools:** Estimate your child's future care expenses, including healthcare and daily living costs. Utilize financial instruments like Special Needs Trusts, which can hold assets while safeguarding eligibility for government benefits.
- **Life Insurance and Investments:** Consider life insurance to provide financial security for your child in your absence. Explore investment options to build a financial safety net for their future needs.

Seeking Expert Guidance

Professional guidance empowers informed decision-making.

- **Financial Advisors with Special Needs Expertise:** Consult a financial advisor familiar with special needs planning. They can help you understand available benefits and create a comprehensive financial plan.
- **Estate Planning and Disability Law Attorneys:** An attorney specializing in estate planning and disability law can assist in drafting legal documents like wills and trusts specific to your child's needs.

- **Recommendations from Medical Professionals:** Seek recommendations for qualified professionals from your child's doctors or therapists.
- **Organization and Preparation:** Gather relevant documents before consultations to ensure a productive exchange with your advisors.

Estate planning and financial security are crucial for the future well-being of your child with CP. By creating a will and potentially setting up a special needs trust, exploring financial strategies, and seeking professional guidance, you can contribute to a secure and fulfilling future for your child.

Remember, proactive planning demonstrates your unwavering love and commitment to ensuring they receive the care and support they need to thrive throughout their life's journey.

11. BUILDING RESILIENCE AS A FAMILY

Coping with Stress and Managing Difficult Emotions

Raising a child with Cerebral Palsy (CP) is a journey filled with love, immense pride, and undeniable challenges.

This section explores the potential sources of stress for parents and siblings, delves into healthy coping mechanisms, and emphasizes the importance of seeking support from others.

Sources of Stress for Families

The weight of caring for a child with CP can manifest in various ways.

- **Parental Stress:** Parents may feel overwhelmed by the demands of caregiving, burdened by financial anxieties about the future, and experience strain in their relationship due to the additional responsibilities.
- **Sibling Challenges:** Siblings may experience feelings of isolation, frustration resulting from additional responsibilities, or a sense of being left out due to the increased attention required by their sibling with CP.

These stressors can manifest physically through headaches, emotionally through anxiety, and behaviorally through academic decline. Recognizing these signs is crucial for intervening and facilitating better stress management within the family.

Building Resilience

Prioritizing self-care empowers families to navigate the challenges.

- **Shared Activities and Exercise:** Engaging in activities like walks or playing in the park together can provide stress relief and strengthen family bonds.
- **Relaxation Techniques:** Techniques like meditation and deep breathing can promote calmness and emotional well-being for both parents and siblings.
- **Prioritizing Basic Needs:** Getting adequate sleep, maintaining a healthy diet, and engaging in hobbies are essential for maintaining emotional and physical resilience.
- **Seeking Support:** Asking for help from family, friends, or therapists demonstrates strength and allows for a more balanced distribution of responsibilities.
- **Open Communication:** For siblings, open communication about CP with parents, quality time with both parents, and pursuing their own activities are crucial for managing emotions.
- **Support Groups:** Connecting with other families through support groups allows siblings to feel understood and share experiences with peers facing similar challenges.

The Power of Shared Experiences

Finding a support system is vital for navigating the complexities of raising a child with CP.

- **Connecting with Others:** Support groups provide a safe space to share experiences, receive advice, and feel a sense of belonging among families who understand the unique challenges.
- **Locating Support:** Support groups can be found at hospitals, disability organizations, online forums, or even through social media platforms.
- **Openness and Shared Successes:** Active listening, sharing experiences openly, and celebrating each other's successes strengthens the support network and fosters a sense of community.

- **Sibling-Specific Support:** Support groups specifically for siblings of children with CP can address their unique challenges and anxieties.

Raising a child with CP requires immense strength and resilience. By acknowledging the potential stressors, implementing healthy coping mechanisms, and actively seeking support from others, families can navigate the challenges and celebrate the joys of this unique journey. Remember, you are not alone. Together, families can build a strong support system that empowers them to provide the best possible care for their loved one with CP while fostering resilience and well-being for all members of the family.

Importance of Self-Care for Parents & Siblings

Raising a child with Cerebral Palsy (CP) is a journey filled with immense love, unwavering dedication, and undeniable challenges.

This section explores the importance of self-care for parents and siblings, emphasizing the analogy of an airplane oxygen mask and highlighting strategies for making time for personal well-being while navigating the demands of caring for a child with CP.

Prioritizing Your Own Needs

Imagine an airplane experiencing turbulence: the safety instructions remind us to secure our own oxygen mask before assisting others. Similarly, in the context of raising a child with CP, prioritizing self-care is not selfish; it is essential for ensuring the well-being of the entire family.

- **Addressing Physical and Mental Health:** Seeking support through respite care allows for much-needed breaks. Techniques like yoga or meditation can promote relaxation and emotional well-being. Maintaining a healthy diet, getting enough sleep, and engaging in exercise are crucial for physical health, which directly impacts mental well-being.

- **Seeking Professional Support:** Do not hesitate to seek help from a therapist if you feel overwhelmed. Talking through challenges and developing coping mechanisms can empower you to navigate difficult emotions.
- **Connecting with Others:** Connecting with other parents of children with CP through support groups or social activities fosters a sense of community and allows for sharing experiences and advice.

Making Time for Activities that Bring Joy

Finding moments for personal fulfillment is crucial for maintaining resilience.

- **Planning and Scheduling:** Schedule time for activities you enjoy, whether it is reading, going for a walk, or pursuing a hobby. This proactive approach ensures time for self-care amidst busy schedules.
- **Delegation and Collaboration:** Do not be afraid to ask for help from your partner, family, or friends. Delegating chores and responsibilities allows for breaks and fosters a sense of shared responsibility within the family. Involving siblings in age-appropriate ways can strengthen family bonds.
- **Finding Pockets of Time:** Self-care does not require extensive time commitments. Even short moments of mindfulness or listening to music can provide a much-needed mental break.

Raising a child with CP is a demanding yet rewarding journey. By prioritizing self-care, utilizing available support systems, and carving out time for personal well-being, parents and siblings can ensure they have the physical and emotional strength to provide the best care for their loved one with CP and maintain a healthy and happy family unit.

Remember, a well-rested and resilient family is better equipped to handle the challenges and celebrate the triumphs that come with raising a child with CP.

Finding Support Groups & Respite Care Options

Raising a child with Cerebral Palsy (CP) is a journey filled with both immense love and significant challenges.

This section explores the importance of finding support groups, participating in online communities, and utilizing respite care options, all crucial aspects of building a support network that empowers parents to navigate this unique path.

Locating Support Groups

No parent should walk this path alone. Connecting with other parents facing similar challenges fosters a sense of community and shared understanding.

- **Seeking Professional Recommendations:** Start by asking your child's doctors or therapists about local support groups. Their expertise can connect you with resources tailored to your specific needs.
- **National Organizations and Online Resources:** Explore online resources offered by national CP organizations. These resources often provide listings of local support groups.
- **Expanding the Search:** Consider checking with local government agencies or disability law specialists for additional support networks in your area.

- **Finding the Right Fit:** Once you find a group, reach out and ask questions to ensure it aligns with your needs and offers a comfortable environment for sharing and learning.

Engaging with Online Communities

The virtual world offers a wealth of support for parents of children with CP.

- **Identifying Your Needs:** Before joining an online community, consider what you seek – a space to share experiences, discover resources, or connect with others for emotional support.
- **Platform Selection:** Choose an online platform you're comfortable with, such as social media groups, dedicated forums, or support group websites with online branches.
- **Netiquette and Respect:** Familiarize yourself with the community's guidelines and introduce yourself thoughtfully. Practice respectful online communication, actively share your own experiences, and ask questions to learn from others.
- **Boundaries and Safety:** Establish healthy online boundaries. Be cautious with personal information, utilize privacy settings, and be wary of misinformation.
- **Maximizing Engagement:** Utilize search functions to find relevant discussions, like and share helpful posts, and consider using private messages for more personal conversations.

Respite Care and Available Services

Taking breaks is essential for maintaining a healthy family dynamic.

- **Respite Care Options:** Respite care provides temporary relief from caregiving duties. This can involve in-home care or specialized programs for short-term stays.

- **Benefits of Respite Care:** Respite care allows for stress reduction, improved well-being for parents, and ultimately, strengthens family bonds.
- **Finding Respite Resources:** Explore options by talking to your child's doctor, contacting disability organizations, checking your health insurance coverage, or researching government programs that offer respite services.
- **Building a Support System:** Consider additional services beyond respite care, such as therapies, support groups, family counseling, or parent training programs. Do not hesitate to seek help from professionals.

Building a Network of Family and Friends

A strong support network extends beyond professional resources.

- **Open Communication:** Have open conversations with family and friends about your needs, whether emotional support or practical help with daily tasks.
- **Delegation and Collaboration:** Identify individual strengths within your network and delegate tasks accordingly. This can include childcare, meal preparation, or errands.
- **Expanding the Circle:** Consider connecting with other parents facing similar experiences to share perspectives and build meaningful connections.
- **Building with Patience:** Remember, building a strong network takes time and effort. Be patient with yourself and those around you.

Raising a child with CP is a journey demanding immense resilience and a strong support system. By actively seeking out support groups, engaging with online communities, exploring respite care options, and fostering a network of family and friends, parents can build a foundation of support that allows them to navigate uncertainty with strength and provide the best possible care for their child. Remember, you are not alone.

Maintaining Strong Family Relationships

Raising a child with Cerebral Palsy (CP) presents a unique set of challenges, but it can also be a journey overflowing with love and pride. This section explores strategies for maintaining strong family relationships, emphasizing the importance of quality time, open communication, celebrating achievements, and fostering a supportive family unit.

Prioritizing Quality Time

Carving out time for shared experiences strengthens the family bond.

- **Short but Meaningful Moments:** Even brief periods of shared laughter, a game night, or a simple conversation can create lasting memories.
- **Scheduling Family Activities:** Plan activities that cater to everyone's interests and abilities. Be flexible and adapt as needed to ensure inclusion for your child with CP.
- **Exploring Sensory Play and Creative Activities:** Sensory play, arts and crafts, or even outdoor adventures can be engaging and enjoyable for the whole family.
- **Memories Over Materialism:** Focus on creating shared experiences and memories rather than expensive outings.

Open Sharing of Feelings

Open communication is the cornerstone of a strong family unit.

- **Creating Safe Spaces for Dialogue:** Establish regular times for open and honest conversations where everyone feels comfortable sharing their feelings and experiences.

- **Honesty and Shared Celebrations:** Be truthful about your child's CP, and celebrate their achievements as a family. Encourage questions and address any concerns openly.
- **Validation and Support:** Acknowledge and validate each other's emotions. Offer support and work together to find solutions to challenges.
- **Including Your Child (When Appropriate):** As your child with CP matures, consider involving them in discussions about their condition to promote self-advocacy.

Recognition and Encouragement

Celebrating achievements fosters confidence and strengthens family connections.

- **Tailored Celebrations:** Choose activities that align with your child's age and interests. Involve siblings and other family members to make celebrations more inclusive.
- **Progress and Effort:** Acknowledge the effort and progress your child makes, not just major milestones. This reinforces positive behavior and motivation.
- **Creating Traditions:** Develop celebratory traditions for achievements, promoting a sense of shared joy and accomplishment.
- **Acknowledging Everyone's Contributions:** Recognize the efforts of everyone involved in your child's care, including yourself and other family members. Simple gestures of appreciation go a long way.

Building a Supportive Family Unit

A strong family unit provides a vital foundation for a child with CP.

- **Open Dialogue and Respectful Communication:** Maintain open and honest communication with all family members, including your child. Listen actively and address concerns with respect.
- **Educating the Family:** Educate your family about CP to foster understanding and empathy. Respect everyone's individual needs and limitations.
- **Shared Responsibilities:** Distribute caregiving tasks and responsibilities among family members based on their abilities. Do not hesitate to seek additional help when needed.
- **Maintaining Optimism and Shared Humor:** Maintain a positive outlook and celebrate achievements, big and small. Do not be afraid to find humor in everyday situations.
- **Connecting with Others and Seeking Resources:** Connect with other families facing similar challenges and explore community resources for support and guidance.

Raising a child with CP is a journey demanding strength, resilience, and a strong family bond. By prioritizing quality time, fostering open communication, celebrating achievements, and building a supportive family unit, you can create an environment where your child feels loved, understood, and empowered to thrive. Remember, the love and support of your family is one of the greatest gifts you can offer your child with CP.

Celebrating Achievements and Milestones

Raising a child with Cerebral Palsy (CP) is a beautiful and complex melody, filled with moments of triumph and passages that require adaptation.

This section explores the importance of celebrating achievements and milestones, focusing on recognizing progress, highlighting strengths and abilities, finding joy in everyday moments, and envisioning a bright future for your child.

Recognizing Progress, Not Perfection

Celebrating a child with CP is about acknowledging their unique path.

- **Shifting the Focus:** Move the spotlight from achieving perfection to appreciating every step forward. Highlight even small improvements in abilities.
- **Applauding Effort and Skills:** Recognize and celebrate the effort behind accomplishments, such as mastering utensil use or utilizing a communication device.
- **Bridging the Gap with Family:** Share updates with relatives through pictures or videos. Provide simple explanations of the challenges your child overcomes.
- **Fostering a Supportive Environment:** Organize family gatherings focused on celebrating achievements. Utilize positive and encouraging language to motivate your child.
- **Embracing the Journey:** Remember, progress is not always linear. Celebrating each milestone, big or small, creates a supportive environment for your child to thrive.

Celebrating Abilities

A child with CP possesses a unique set of strengths waiting to be celebrated.

- **Beyond Limitations:** Move beyond focusing solely on challenges. Identify and celebrate your child's strengths, such as creativity or unwavering determination.
- **Sharing Stories of Growth:** With family members, share stories that highlight your child's progress and positive personality traits.
- **Activities that Empower:** Plan activities that allow your child to shine, whether it is reading aloud or showcasing musical talents.

- **Encouraging Self-Advocacy:** Empower your child to speak up for themselves and make choices that capitalize on their strengths.
- **Building Confidence:** Offer praise for effort and display achievements around the house to create a confidence-boosting environment.

Finding the Melody in Everyday Moments

Moments of joy can be found throughout the journey with CP.

- **Celebrating Strengths, Big and Small:** Recognize and celebrate your child's strengths, from major achievements to seemingly simple victories like tying their shoes.
- **Shared Activities and Sensory Play:** Engage in fun activities together, tailoring games and sensory experiences to your child's interests and abilities.
- **Strengthening Family Bonds:** Involve the entire family in daily tasks and share moments of happiness to strengthen your bond.
- **Prioritizing Self-Care:** Remember to take care of yourself too. Schedule time for activities that bring you joy.
- **Finding the Positive:** By focusing on the positive aspects of your journey and creating joyful memories together, you can cultivate a sense of happiness within your family.

Composing a Future Filled with Potential

A diagnosis of CP does not define a child's future potential.

- **Strengths as the Foundation:** Build upon your child's strengths as the foundation for their future.
- **Celebrating Achievements:** Recognize and celebrate their accomplishments, fostering a sense of pride and confidence.

- **Positive Language and Open Communication:** Utilize positive language when discussing your child's future and maintain open communication within the family.
- **Building a Support System:** Connect with other families facing similar challenges and explore community resources to build a supportive network.
- **Embracing Individuality:** Every child is unique. Embrace your child's individual journey and celebrate their differences.
- **Creating a Positive Environment:** By creating a positive and inclusive environment, you empower your child to reach their full potential and achieve a fulfilling future.

Raising a child with CP is a journey filled with unique challenges and extraordinary triumphs. By celebrating achievements, big and small, focusing on strengths and abilities, finding joy in everyday moments, and envisioning a bright future, you can create a beautiful symphony of love, support, and empowerment that allows your child to thrive.

Remember, every note in your child's song is worth celebrating.

12. SIBLINGS ON THE JOURNEY

The Unique Role of Siblings

The presence of a sibling with Cerebral Palsy (CP) can introduce complexities into the lives of other children in the family.

This section explores strategies for addressing potential feelings of jealousy or isolation, fostering a strong sibling bond, and encouraging empathy and understanding.

Acknowledging and Addressing Difficult Emotions

It is crucial to create a safe space for your child without CP to express their feelings.

- **Open Communication:** Encourage open and honest communication. Validate their emotions and create a space where they can express feelings of jealousy, resentment, or isolation without judgment.
- **One-on-One Time:** Schedule regular one-on-one activities with your child. Demonstrate your love and value for them as an individual.
- **Reassurance and Empathy Building:** Reassure them that your love is constant, even when your attention may shift due to their sibling's needs. Help them understand their sibling's perspective, fostering empathy and understanding.

Building Understanding and Connection

Fostering a strong sibling bond strengthens the family unit.

- **Open Dialogue:** Maintain open conversations about CP. Answer questions honestly and acknowledge their feelings.

- **Celebrating Individuality:** Celebrate each child's unique strengths and talents. Plan activities that cater to their individual interests while allowing for shared participation.
- **Empathy Through Inclusion:** Consider involving your child without CP in therapy sessions or doctor's appointments (age-appropriately) to build understanding and empathy. Celebrate milestones achieved by both children.
- **Positive Reinforcement:** Acknowledge and praise acts of kindness or support your child without CP shows towards their sibling.
- **Nurturing Individual Connections:** Schedule quality one-on-one time with each child, strengthening individual relationships within the family.

Shared Experiences and Respectful Boundaries

Shared activities foster connection while respecting individuality.

- **Finding Common Ground:** Identify activities that all siblings can enjoy together, like adapted sports or games. Focus on fun and participation, not competition.
- **Celebrating Individual Achievements:** Acknowledge and celebrate each child's unique accomplishments, whether it is mastering a therapeutic exercise or excelling in a hobby.
- **Teamwork with Respect:** Encourage teamwork during shared activities, while still offering opportunities for individual pursuits.
- **Praising Inclusion:** Recognize and acknowledge moments of collaboration or inclusion between siblings.

Building a strong sibling bond takes time, patience, and consistent effort. By addressing difficult emotions, fostering empathy, and encouraging shared activities, we can help siblings navigate the complexities of having a brother or sister with CP. This ultimately leads to a stronger family unit, where each child feels loved, valued, and supported for who they are.

Communication and Open Dialogue

The presence of Cerebral Palsy (CP) in a family can introduce complexities into sibling relationships. Open and honest communication is crucial for fostering understanding, empathy, and a strong bond between siblings.

This section explores strategies for discussing CP in an age-appropriate way, creating a safe space for siblings to express their emotions, and ultimately, encouraging open communication that builds a supportive relationship.

Age-Appropriate Communication about CP

Discussing CP with siblings requires tailoring the conversation to their age and understanding.

- **Choosing the Right Moment:** Select a calm and relaxed environment where everyone feels comfortable talking openly.
- **Simple Explanations:** Explain CP in clear and simple terms. Consider phrases like "the brain sends messages to the body differently," highlighting the need for extra support with mobility or communication.
- **Age-Appropriate Examples:** Use relatable examples that resonate with their age and experiences to enhance understanding.
- **A Safe Space for Emotions:** Acknowledge that their feelings of confusion or frustration are valid, and reassure them that you are always available to listen.
- **Positive Language and Highlighting Strengths:** Focus on their sibling's strengths and talents, framing CP in a positive light.
- **Encouraging Questions and Honesty:** Promote open communication by encouraging questions and honest expression

of their feelings. Consider reading age-appropriate books about siblings with CP together to foster further understanding.

- **Sibling Participation (when comfortable):** If your child with CP feels comfortable, involve them in the conversation to share their experiences and perspectives.

Creating a Platform for Emotional Expression

A safe space allows siblings to openly express their emotions.

- **Open Door Policy:** Reassure them that you are always available to talk, creating a safe space for open communication.
- **Active Listening and Validation:** Dedicate individual time to each sibling, actively listening to their concerns and validating their feelings without judgment.
- **Creative Expression:** Encourage them to express their emotions creatively through drawing, writing, or playing music.
- **Shared Experiences:** Share stories of other families with siblings navigating similar situations to foster a sense of belonging and understanding.
- **Celebrating Individuality:** Acknowledge and celebrate what makes each child special, highlighting their unique strengths and personalities.
- **Shared Activities and Individual Pursuits:** Find activities enjoyable for everyone, while respecting individual interests and allowing dedicated time for each child's hobbies.

Fostering a Supportive and Open Relationship

Open communication paves the way for a strong bond between siblings.

- **Unconditional Support:** Reassure both children that they can always talk to you openly about anything, without fear of judgment.

- **Empathy Through Understanding:** Encourage activities that foster empathy, allowing siblings to see the world from each other's perspectives.
- **Celebrating Differences and Similarities:** Celebrate what makes each of them special, acknowledging both their differences and the joys of being siblings.
- **Shared Experiences and Adapted Activities:** Engage in activities they can both enjoy, even if adaptations are needed for your child with CP.
- **Positive Reinforcement:** Acknowledge and praise acts of kindness and support between siblings, strengthening their bond.
- **Openness and Patience:** Be open about your child's condition and continue to have conversations as they grow and their understanding deepens.

Communication is the cornerstone of a strong sibling relationship, especially when one child has CP. By creating a safe space for open dialogue, fostering empathy, and encouraging honest expression of emotions, we can help siblings build a supportive and loving bond that transcends the challenges of CP. This open communication will allow them to navigate life's journey together, celebrating their individuality while cherishing the unique connection they share as siblings.

Supporting Sibling Development

The presence of a sibling with Cerebral Palsy (CP) can impact the development of other children in the family.

This section explores strategies for addressing potential delays and social struggles, providing resources to support individual needs, and encouraging involvement in activities outside of sibling care.

Addressing Potential Challenges

It is crucial to acknowledge and address any challenges siblings may face.

- **Open Communication:** Maintain open communication channels. Allow siblings to express feelings of frustration or isolation without judgment. Reassure them of your unconditional love and support.
- **Validating Emotions:** Acknowledge that feelings of being left out or unsure are normal. Help them understand and navigate these emotions in a healthy way.
- **Individualized Attention:** Dedicate time for each child to pursue their own interests and talents. Celebrate their unique achievements and strengths.
- **Building Connections:** Encourage interaction between siblings to foster understanding and empathy. Activities that promote shared experiences can strengthen their bond.
- **Building a Support Network:** If a sibling struggles significantly, consider seeking professional support from a counselor specializing in families with children with disabilities.

Support for Individual Needs

Meeting each child's unique needs is vital for their development.
- **Open Dialogue:** Talk openly about their feelings and validate their frustrations. Understanding their perspective allows for tailored support.
- **Quality Time and Recognition:** Dedicate individual time for each child, engaging in activities they enjoy. Celebrate their achievements, boosting their confidence and sense of self.
- **Shared Experiences with Adjustments:** Find activities that everyone can enjoy together, even if adaptations are needed. This fosters a sense of inclusion and belonging.

- **Appreciating Differences:** Encourage siblings to appreciate each other's strengths and unique qualities. This fosters a sense of respect and strengthens the bond.
- **Support Groups and Resources:** Explore support groups or programs specifically for siblings of children with disabilities. These resources can provide valuable peer connection and guidance.
- **Professional Support:** If a sibling experiences significant challenges, seeking professional help from a counselor familiar with families like yours can be beneficial.

Encouraging Personal Growth Beyond Sibling Care

A healthy balance is crucial for sibling development.

- **One-on-One Time:** Schedule dedicated one-on-one time with your child without CP to demonstrate their importance as an individual.
- **Exploring Interests:** Help them explore and pursue their interests by enrolling them in clubs or groups related to their hobbies.
- **Fostering Independence:** Support their participation in their hobbies by providing transportation, equipment, or any resources they may need.
- **Celebrating Achievements:** Recognize and celebrate their accomplishments in their chosen activities, fostering a sense of pride and motivation.
- **Balancing Responsibilities:** Encourage them to help with their sibling's care when appropriate. However, ensure they have time to focus on their own goals and interests.

Having a sibling with CP presents unique challenges and opportunities. By fostering open communication, providing targeted support, and encouraging individual development, we can help siblings navigate these challenges, build strong bonds, and thrive as individuals while enriching the lives of their brother or sister with CP.

13. BUILDING A FULFILLING LIFE

Identifying Your Child's Passions and Interests

Every child, including those with Cerebral Palsy (CP), possesses unique talents and interests.

This section explores strategies for parents to help their children with CP embark on a journey of discovery, identifying passions that ignite their curiosity and foster a sense of purpose.

Encouraging Exploration and Fostering Discovery

The key to uncovering a child's passions lies in creating a nurturing environment that encourages exploration.

- **Accessible Activities:** Choose activities that are engaging and adapted for your child's physical limitations. Consider using assistive technology or modified materials to ensure participation.
- **Variety is Key:** Explore a diverse range of activities, from music and art to science experiments. Expose your child to different experiences to discover areas that spark their enthusiasm.
- **Celebrating Effort:** Focus on the joy of participation and effort rather than achieving perfection. Celebrate their attempts and encourage them to discover their unique strengths.
- **Learning in Everyday Moments:** Integrate learning opportunities into daily activities. Observe what captures their attention during everyday routines and build upon their interests.

Participation and Personalized Exploration

Once you begin to identify potential interests, provide opportunities for further exploration.

- **Building on Interests:** Support your child in delving deeper into activities they show enthusiasm for. Enroll them in adapted programs, like sports teams or art therapy workshops, catering to children with CP.
- **Community Resources:** Connect with local organizations or online communities that specialize in activities for children with CP.
- **Focus on Fun:** Remember, enjoyment is paramount. Celebrate their participation and be their biggest supporter, fostering a positive attitude towards exploration.

Embracing Purpose and Fulfillment

A child's life with CP can be enriched and empowered through a focus on their passions.

- **Nurturing Interests:** Encourage and support them in developing their talents and interests, be it music, art, sports, or anything that ignites their spirit.
- **Celebrating Milestones:** Acknowledge their achievements, big or small, to fuel their motivation and sense of accomplishment.
- **Social Connection:** Help them build friendships and connect with communities that share their passions.
- **Developing Purpose:** Explore volunteer opportunities or ways they can contribute to their community, fostering a sense of purpose beyond their limitations.
- **Empowerment and Choice:** Encourage independence by allowing them to make choices and participate in activities as much as possible.
- **Role Models of Triumph:** Share stories of successful individuals with CP to inspire them and demonstrate the limitless possibilities within their reach.

CP may present challenges, but it does not define a child's potential. By creating a stimulating environment, providing opportunities for exploration, and celebrating their unique talents, we can help children with CP discover their passions, leading to a life filled with purpose, joy, and a sense of accomplishment. This journey of discovery requires patience, support, and a focus on fostering the flame of their inner passion. By nurturing these interests, we empower children with CP to embrace a fulfilling life filled with their unique contributions to the world.

Promoting Independence and Self-Advocacy

Cerebral Palsy (CP) presents challenges to a child's development of independence and self-advocacy skills. However, with patience, support, and the right strategies, children with CP can blossom into self-assured individuals capable of navigating their world and expressing their needs effectively.

This section explores methods for promoting age-appropriate decision-making, teaching self-advocacy tools, and empowering children with CP to navigate their environment with confidence.

Building the Foundation for Independence

Encouraging a sense of autonomy starts with small yet significant steps.

- **Empowering Choices:** Offer age-appropriate choices, allowing your child to make decisions within set parameters. Celebrate their choices, no matter how small, fostering a sense of control.
- **Breaking Down Tasks:** Break down complex tasks into manageable steps, providing guidance and support as they learn to complete them independently. Gradually reduce assistance as their confidence grows.

- **Adaptive Tools and Techniques:** Utilize assistive technology and adapted tools to make everyday activities easier, promoting a sense of self-reliance.
- **Celebrating Progress:** Acknowledge and celebrate even small steps towards independence. Positive reinforcement fuels motivation and a desire to achieve further independence.

Equipping Them for Self-Advocacy

Effective communication is vital for self-advocacy. Here is how to empower your child.

- **Communication Tools:** Start with simple tools like picture cards or gestures to communicate basic needs and emotions. Gradually introduce more complex methods of expression.
- **The Power of Choice:** Encourage your child to make choices and express their preferences whenever possible. Role-playing scenarios can help them practice self-advocacy in different situations.
- **Assistive Technology and Therapy:** Explore assistive technology or speech therapy to enhance communication skills and empower them to express themselves clearly.
- **Open Communication:** Maintain open and supportive communication channels. Listen actively to their feelings and validate their frustrations.

Empowering Exploration & Building Confidence

A confident child is more likely to embrace independence. Here is how to foster confidence.

- **Breaking Down Challenges:** Break down tasks into achievable steps, celebrating each accomplishment and building a sense of mastery.

- **Promoting Mobility:** Utilize physical therapy and assistive technology to improve mobility, allowing them to explore their surroundings more independently.
- **Strength-Based Approach:** Focus on your child's strengths and encourage them to build upon their abilities. This fosters a sense of self-belief and confidence.
- **Problem-Solving Skills:** Involve your child in everyday problem-solving and decision-making. This equips them with the skills to navigate challenges independently.
- **Peer Interaction:** Encourage interaction with peers, promoting social skills and a sense of belonging within their environment.

By fostering a supportive environment that promotes decision-making, equips them with self-advocacy tools, and empowers them to navigate their surroundings, we can help children with CP build the wings they need to soar towards independence and a life filled with confidence and self-expression.

Remember, this journey is a marathon, not a sprint. With unwavering support and a focus on progress, we can empower children with CP to reach their full potential and embrace a fulfilling life.

Fostering a Positive Future Outlook

A diagnosis of Cerebral Palsy (CP) can raise concerns about a child's future. However, with a focus on setting realistic goals, fostering a vision of possibility, and connecting with positive role models, we can empower children with CP to embrace a future rich in opportunity and achievement.

This section explores strategies for setting achievable goals, envisioning a fulfilling future, and finding inspiration in the success stories of others in the CP community.

Celebrating Milestones on the Path to Success

Goal setting is crucial for fostering confidence and a sense of accomplishment. Here is how to ensure a successful journey.

- **Realistic Benchmarks:** Collaborate with therapists to establish achievable goals that align with your child's unique abilities and development.
- **Breaking Down Barriers:** Break down large goals into smaller, manageable tasks, celebrating each completed step and encouraging further progress.
- **The Power of Recognition:** Celebrate achievements, big or small, with positive reinforcement like rewards, verbal praise, or visual reminders of their progress. Recognition fuels motivation and a sense of accomplishment.

Envisioning Possibilities and Unleashing Potential

Looking beyond limitations fosters a positive outlook on the future.

- **Strengths-Based Approach:** Focus on your child's strengths, interests, and talents. Celebrate their achievements and use empowering language that highlights their capabilities.
- **Dream Big:** Encourage them to explore diverse activities and dream big about their future. A positive outlook opens doors to a world of possibilities.
- **Building Confidence:** Celebrate every success, no matter how small, to boost their confidence and keep them motivated on their journey.

Finding Inspiration in the CP Community

Surrounding your child with positive influences can be incredibly empowering.

- **Role Models of Resilience:** Connect with support groups, online communities, and disability organizations to find inspiring stories of individuals with CP who are thriving in various fields.
- **Shared Journeys and Successes:** Share stories of successful individuals with CP and discuss how these stories relate to your child's own goals and interests. Highlight the similarities between your child and these role models, fostering a sense of shared journey and achievable dreams.
- **Celebrating Collective Achievements:** Celebrate the achievements of others in the CP community, creating a sense of belonging and fostering inspiration for your child's own future.

A child with CP faces unique challenges, but their potential for a fulfilling life is limitless. By setting realistic goals, fostering a vision of a hopeful future, and connecting with positive role models, we can build bridges of hope that empower children with CP to embrace their potential and confidently navigate the road to a bright and fulfilling future.

Remember, with unwavering support, a focus on their strengths, and a belief in their dreams, children with CP can achieve great things and leave their unique mark on the world.

Setting realistic goals & celebrating achievements

As a parent of a child with CP, it is important to set small, achievable goals and celebrate each step of progress. Break down bigger goals into smaller tasks, and focus on what your child can do. Work with their therapists to set realistic goals that match their abilities and development. Celebrate every achievement, whether big or small, with rewards, verbal praise, or visual reminders of their progress.

Remember, it is about celebrating their journey and encouraging them along the way, no matter how small the steps may seem.

Envisioning a fulfilling future & focusing on possibilities

As a parent of a child with CP, it is important to see beyond limitations and focus on their strengths and interests. Celebrate every achievement, big or small, to boost their confidence and keep them motivated. Use empowering language that highlights their capabilities instead of their limitations. Encourage them to explore different activities and dream big about their future. With the right support and belief in their potential, your child can achieve great things and lead a fulfilling life.

Connecting with positive role models & success stories

You can find inspiring stories and role models for your child with CP through support groups, online communities, social media, and disability organizations. Look for stories of people with CP who are succeeding in different areas of life, like sports, art, or career. Share these stories with your child and discuss how they relate to their own goals and interests. Focus on similarities between your child and these role models, and celebrate their achievements along the way. These connections can inspire and motivate your child to pursue their dreams and see the possibilities for their future.

14. EVERYDAY CHALLENGES

Discipline and Behavior Management

Cerebral Palsy (CP) presents unique challenges for children and their parents. Traditional discipline techniques may not be as effective, requiring a more nuanced approach.

This section explores key strategies for successful discipline and behavior management for children with CP, emphasizing positive reinforcement, clear communication, and consistency.

Adapting Traditional Techniques

Children with CP may struggle to understand complex instructions or communicate their needs effectively. Here is how to adapt traditional approaches.

- **Focus on Positive Reinforcement:** Instead of punishment, prioritize praise for good behavior. This creates a positive association with desired actions and motivates your child to repeat them.
- **Clear Communication:** Use simple, concise language and pair instructions with visual aids like pictures or charts. Gestures and facial expressions can further enhance communication clarity.
- **Understanding Limitations:** Consider any physical limitations your child might have and be patient during communication. Frustration with limitations can sometimes lead to behavioral issues.

Building a Positive Approach

Effective behavior management for children with CP requires a positive and consistent approach.

- **Understanding Behavior:** Sometimes, challenging behavior stems from communication difficulties, sensory overload, or frustration caused by physical limitations. Addressing these underlying issues can help prevent behavioral issues.
- **Positive Language:** Set expectations using clear, calm language. Avoid yelling or harsh words, as these can escalate the situation.
- **Consistency is Key:** Collaborate with therapists and caregivers to establish a consistent routine and behavior management plan. Everyone involved – parents, teachers, therapists – should adhere to the same approach for optimal results.

The Power of Positive Reinforcement

Rewards and positive reinforcement are powerful tools for encouraging desired behavior in children with CP.

- **Praise and Recognition:** Acknowledge and celebrate your child's achievements, no matter how small. This positive reinforcement reinforces desired behaviors.
- **Tailored Rewards:** Choose rewards that motivate your child, such as extra playtime with a favorite toy or participating in a preferred activity.
- **Patience and Encouragement:** Learning takes time. Be patient, offer consistent encouragement, and smile to create a positive learning environment.

Seeking Support

Remember, you are not alone. There are resources available to help you on this journey.

- **Professional Guidance:** Do not hesitate to seek help from therapists or specialists who can provide guidance and support in developing a personalized behavior management plan.

- **Connecting with Others:** Connecting with other parents raising children with CP can be a valuable source of support, advice, and shared experiences.

By adapting traditional discipline techniques, building a positive and consistent approach, and utilizing the power of positive reinforcement, you can effectively manage your child's behavior and help them thrive despite the challenges of CP. The journey may not always be smooth, but with patience, understanding, and the right support systems in place, you can guide your child towards a future filled with positive experiences and successful interactions.

Fostering Harmony between Siblings

The arrival of a new sibling is a joyous occasion, but for the existing child, it can also stir up feelings of jealousy and confusion. These emotions are amplified when a sibling has Cerebral Palsy (CP).

This section explores strategies for addressing sibling rivalry, promoting cooperation, and encouraging empathy between siblings, fostering a strong bond despite the challenges of CP.

Acknowledging Emotions

Addressing sibling jealousy is crucial for building a positive relationship.

- **Validate Feelings:** Acknowledge that it is normal to feel jealous or frustrated sometimes. Let siblings know it is okay to express their emotions openly, creating a safe space for them to talk.
- **Quality Time:** Spend dedicated time with each child individually. This shows both children they are valued and creates space for unique connections.

Building a Foundation for Cooperation

Finding common ground is key to encouraging cooperation and shared play.

- **Shared Activities:** Look for activities both siblings can enjoy, adapting them as needed. Building with blocks (using larger ones for the child with CP) or listening to music are examples.
- **Teamwork and Shared Strengths:** Create games that require teamwork, celebrating each child's strengths and assigning supportive roles during playtime.
- **Realistic Expectations:** Playtime might look different when one child has CP. Set realistic expectations and acknowledge that adjustments might be needed.
- **One-on-One Time:** Balance shared activities with dedicated one-on-one time for each child. This caters to individual needs and interests.

Cultivating Empathy and Understanding

Empathy is the cornerstone of a strong sibling bond. Here is how to nurture it.

- **Open Communication:** Create a safe space for open communication where both children can express their feelings without judgement.
- **Role-Playing Games:** Use role-playing games to help siblings understand each other's perspectives. This fosters empathy for the challenges of CP.
- **"I" Statements:** Encourage children to express their feelings using "I" statements like "I feel frustrated when..." This promotes clear communication of needs.
- **Celebrating Differences:** Celebrate what makes each child unique and special. This fosters acceptance and understanding.

Building a strong relationship between siblings takes time, patience, and continuous effort. By acknowledging emotions, promoting cooperation, and cultivating empathy, parents can help siblings overcome challenges related to CP and lay the foundation for a loving and supportive lifelong bond.

Remember, with the right approach, siblings can become each other's greatest allies and sources of encouragement.

Managing Mealtimes and Nutrition

Mealtimes can present unique challenges for children with Cerebral Palsy (CP). Motor skill limitations and coordination difficulties can make eating a frustrating experience for both child and caregiver. However, with a combination of therapy, dietary adjustments, and adaptations, mealtimes can be transformed into safe, nutritious, and even enjoyable events.

This section explores strategies for addressing feeding difficulties, promoting a balanced diet, and adapting mealtimes for safety and independence.

Overcoming Feeding Difficulties

Addressing feeding challenges requires a multi-pronged approach.

- **Understanding the Source:** Consulting with a doctor is the first step. They can identify the specific challenges, such as motor skills limitations or swallowing difficulties.
- **Therapy and Support:** Therapists play a crucial role. Occupational therapists can improve coordination and motor skills, while speech therapists may address swallowing issues.

- **Adaptive Equipment:** Utilizing specialized utensils with weighted grips or angled handles, proper positioning during meals, and tray tables can significantly improve safety and independence.
- **Patience and Consistency:** Therapy exercises need to be practiced consistently at home. Patience is key, as progress might be gradual.
- **Dietary Modifications:** Consider thickened liquids for swallowing difficulties and offer a variety of textures to encourage exploration of food.

Fueling Growth and Development

Ensuring a balanced and nutritious diet is crucial for a child with CP.

- **Variety is Key:** Offer a rainbow of fruits and vegetables, protein sources, and whole grains to ensure a balanced intake of essential nutrients.
- **Hydration Matters:** Encourage regular water intake to prevent dehydration.
- **Involving the Child:** Meal planning and cooking can be a fun way to foster a positive association with food. Let your child participate in age-appropriate ways.
- **Positive Reinforcement:** Maintain a calm and positive atmosphere during mealtimes. Celebrate attempts at new foods, fostering a sense of accomplishment.
- **Seeking Professional Guidance:** Dietitians or therapists can offer personalized advice on creating a healthy meal plan for your child's specific needs.

Empowering Independence

By adapting mealtimes and utensils, we can create opportunities for children with CP to develop independence.

- **Adaptive Utensils:** Experiment with utensils that are easier to hold, like weighted forks or spoons with thicker handles.
- **Ensuring Comfort:** Good posture is vital. Use chairs with proper support and explore tray tables to minimize spills.
- **Food Adaptations:** Cut food into manageable pieces or choose options with softer textures for easier chewing.
- **Patience and Encouragement:** Be patient as your child learns to feed themselves. Positive reinforcement goes a long way.

Mealtimes do not have to be a battleground for children with CP. By addressing feeding difficulties, prioritizing a balanced diet, and adapting mealtimes, we can create safe, positive, and empowering experiences that contribute to their overall health and well-being. With patience, collaboration, and the right support systems in place, mealtimes can become a time for connection, exploration, and joyful interaction for children with CP and their families.

Sleep and Rest

Cerebral Palsy (CP) can disrupt a child's sleep patterns, impacting their overall well-being. Understanding how CP affects sleep is the first step towards creating a calming and restorative sleep environment.

This section explores the sleep challenges associated with CP and delves into strategies for developing healthy sleep routines and addressing sleep disruptions.

Understanding the Disruptions

Several factors related to CP can hinder a child's sleep.

- **Muscle Stiffness and Discomfort:** Tight muscles can make it difficult to find a comfortable sleeping position, leading to restlessness and frequent awakenings.

- **Involuntary Movements:** Children with CP might experience involuntary movements like spasticity, further disrupting sleep.
- **Breathing Difficulties:** Some children with CP have respiratory issues, impacting oxygen levels and causing sleep disturbances.

Promoting Restful Sleep

Creating healthy sleep routines can significantly improve sleep quality for children with CP:

- **Consistent Sleep Schedule:** Establish a consistent bedtime and wake-up time, even on weekends, to regulate the body's natural sleep-wake cycle.
- **Calming Bedtime Routine:** Develop a relaxing bedtime routine that signals to the body it is time to wind down. This could include taking a warm bath, reading a story, or listening to calming music.
- **Comfortable Sleep Environment:** Ensure the bedroom is quiet, dark, and cool; the factors conducive to restful sleep.
- **Addressing Pain:** If pain is a contributing factor, discuss pain management strategies with a doctor. This might involve medication, physiotherapy, or positioning techniques.
- **Promoting Relaxation Techniques:** Encourage daytime exercise to release energy and consider relaxation techniques like deep breathing or gentle stretches before bed.

Addressing Sleep Disruptions

Persistent sleep problems require a more targeted approach.

- **Consulting a Doctor:** Discuss your child's sleep issues with a doctor to rule out any underlying medical conditions.
- **Medication:** In certain cases, medication might be necessary to address specific sleep challenges.

- **Seeking Specialized Help:** A sleep specialist can offer personalized advice and strategies tailored to your child's unique needs.
- **Patience and Consistency:** Developing healthy sleep habits takes time and consistency. Be patient and celebrate small improvements.

Prioritizing sleep is crucial for a child's physical and mental well-being. By understanding how CP affects sleep patterns, creating healthy sleep routines, and addressing disruptions with appropriate strategies, parents can help their child with CP experience a symphony of slumber, fostering a foundation for optimal development and growth.

Remember, collaboration with healthcare professionals is key to achieving restful sleep for your child.

Leisure Activities & Playtime

Cerebral Palsy (CP) may present challenges for a child's playtime experiences. However, with a focus on adapted toys, inclusive activities, and fostering social interaction, playtime can become a fun and enriching experience for both the child with CP and their peers.

This section explores strategies for finding engaging adapted toys, encouraging participation in social activities, and creating inclusive play environments.

Unlocking the World of Play with Adapted Toys

The right toys can spark a child's imagination and promote development. When choosing adapted toys for a child with CP, consider these factor.

- **Matching Interests and Abilities:** Select toys that cater to the child's age, interests, and physical capabilities. Look for features like large buttons or switches for easy grasping.
- **Sensory Exploration:** Toys with different textures, sounds, and lights can stimulate the senses and encourage engagement.
- **Seeking Recommendations:** Therapists and online resources can offer valuable guidance on finding suitable adapted toys.

Embracing Social Activities and Group Play

Social interaction and group play are vital for a child's development. Here is how to encourage participation for children with CP.

- **Finding the Right Fit:** Look for activities that align with the child's interests and abilities. Adapted sports like wheelchair basketball or swimming programs are great options.
- **Building Confidence:** Start with smaller groups and gradually progress to larger ones, fostering confidence and social skills development.
- **Adapting for Inclusion:** Utilize adaptive equipment and modify rules to ensure full participation and enjoyment by all children.
- **Focusing on Fun:** Emphasize the joy of participation over winning.
- **Leading by Example:** Actively participate alongside your child, demonstrating the value of social interaction.
- **Communication and Support:** Communicate the child's needs to activity organizers and celebrate their efforts. Offer unwavering patience and support throughout the process.

Creating Inclusive Play Environments

By making play environments inclusive, we can foster meaningful connections between children with CP and their peers.

- **Similar Activities:** Choose activities that allow for participation by all children, regardless of abilities. Modified games or group activities can be a great option.
- **Focus on Collaboration:** Encourage teamwork and cooperation during playtime, fostering a sense of belonging and shared accomplishment.
- **Celebrating Differences:** Create a space where all children feel valued and appreciated for their unique strengths and abilities.

Playtime is not just about entertainment; it is a crucial element in a child's development. By embracing adapted toys, encouraging participation in social activities, and fostering inclusive play environments, we can unlock a world of possibilities for children with CP. Playtime becomes a bridge to social connection, skill development, and a joyful childhood experience for all children to share.

Technology and Screen Time

Technology has the remarkable potential to transform the lives of children with Cerebral Palsy (CP) by opening doors to communication, learning, and entertainment.

This section explores the benefits of technology in various aspects of a child's life, while emphasizing the importance of healthy screen time habits and finding accessible resources.

Unlocking Communication and Expression

Assistive technology bridges the communication gap for children with CP.

- **Speech-Generating Devices:** These devices provide a voice to children who struggle with speech, empowering them to express themselves and participate in conversations.

- **Video Chat Apps:** Connecting with loved ones becomes easier with video chat apps, fostering social interaction and reducing feelings of isolation.

Enhancing Learning and Development

Technology offers a multitude of educational tools specifically designed for children with CP.

- **Educational Apps and E-readers:** These tools cater to different learning styles and abilities, offering interactive ways to explore various subjects.
- **Special Features:** E-readers with text-to-speech capabilities or adaptations for easier reading enhance the learning experience.

Expanding Entertainment Horizons

Technology keeps children entertained and engaged.

- **Adapted Games:** Games with adapted controls allow children with CP to enjoy the world of gaming, fostering recreation and social interaction with peers.
- **Streaming Services:** Closed captioning on streaming platforms makes movies and shows accessible, providing a source of enjoyment and relaxation.

Finding the Right Fit

When introducing technology, consider these factors.

- **Focus on Needs and Interests:** Prioritize apps and devices that cater to your child's specific needs and interests, ensuring their engagement and enjoyment.

- **Start Simple, Progress Gradually:** Start with simple technology and gradually introduce more complex options as your child's skills develop.

Balance and Safety

While technology offers numerous benefits, establishing healthy screen time limits is crucial.

- **Age-Appropriate Usage:** Consider your child's age, attention span, and physical limitations when determining screen time.
- **Balance with Other Activities:** Encourage a healthy balance between technology use and other activities like playing outdoors or reading.
- **Gradual Reduction:** If your child is used to a lot of screen time, reduce it gradually to promote a more balanced routine.

Parental Controls and Open Communication

Safety is paramount in the digital world.

- **Parental Controls:** Utilize parental controls to filter out inappropriate content and ensure your child's online safety.
- **Open Dialogue:** Discuss online safety with your child and encourage open communication regarding their online activities.
- **Respecting Privacy:** As your child gets older, respect their developing need for privacy while maintaining appropriate supervision.

Finding Accessible Resources

Numerous resources cater to children with CP.

- **Online Resources:** Organizations like the Cerebral Palsy Foundation provide lists of accessible apps and programs.
- **Therapist Recommendations:** Consult your child's therapists for recommendations on technology that aligns with their specific needs.
- **Exploring Options:** Look beyond apps and consider interactive websites, specialized learning materials, and tools like voice commands or special keyboards that make online activities easier.

Technology's potential to empower children with CP is vast. From facilitating communication to enhancing learning and entertainment, it opens up a world of opportunity. By utilizing a balanced approach, prioritizing safety, and finding accessible resources, parents can help their children with CP leverage technology to reach their full potential and thrive in a world increasingly driven by digital connection.

15. ASSISTIVE TECHNOLOGY

Cerebral Palsy (CP) can present challenges for children in communication, mobility, and learning. However, advancements in assistive technology (AT) offer a wealth of tools to empower children with CP and unlock their full potential.

This section explores three key categories of AT: Augmentative and Alternative Communication (AAC) devices, assistive devices for mobility and independence, and computer adaptations and educational software.

Finding Their Voice: AAC Devices

For children with CP who struggle to speak, AAC devices bridge the communication gap. These tools come in various forms, from simple picture boards to sophisticated voice synthesizers and tablet apps. Starting with a simple picture board and gradually progressing to more complex devices is a common approach. Therapists play a crucial role in selecting the appropriate device and teaching parents and children how to use it effectively. AAC empowers children with CP to express themselves, fostering independence, improving communication skills, and aiding their learning journey. Patience, practice, and celebration of milestones are key to a successful AAC journey.

Enhancing Mobility and Independence

Assistive devices for mobility and independence, like walkers, wheelchairs, and standing frames, can significantly improve a child's quality of life. Doctors, therapists, or specialists will recommend the most suitable device based on the child's individual needs. Walkers provide extra support for walking, wheelchairs offer freedom of movement for those who find walking difficult, and standing frames help children practice standing for improved physical development.

These devices allow children with CP to explore their surroundings, participate in activities, and develop their physical abilities. Proper fitting, training on safe device use, and exploring financial assistance programs are crucial considerations for parents.

Learning with Technology

When it comes to learning, technology plays a vital role. For children with CP, computer adaptations and educational software can make a significant difference. Computers can be adapted with features like voice commands or trackballs to make them more accessible. Educational software designed for different ages and learning styles can cater to various needs, from reading comprehension to math skills. Finding engaging and interactive software with features like text-to-speech or simplified controls can enhance a child's learning experience. Therapists and online resources can offer valuable recommendations for software selection. Remember, technology complements traditional learning methods and works best when combined with support from parents, teachers, and therapists.

Choosing the Right Tools

Selecting the right AT for your child with CP involves considering their physical abilities, communication methods, and learning goals. Activities should be chosen based on these factors, fostering the development of new skills. Involving the whole family in engaging activities can create positive learning experiences. When exploring educational options, consult with doctors and teachers, research online resources, and visit schools or therapy centers to find the best fit for your child and family.

Remember, there are numerous resources available to help you navigate the world of AT. Doctors, therapists, and various organizations can guide you in finding the perfect tools to empower your child with CP and help them reach their full potential.

By harnessing the power of assistive technology, children with CP can overcome challenges, embrace new possibilities, and lead fulfilling lives.

16. THE ROLE OF THERAPY

Cerebral Palsy (CP) is a group of neurological disorders affecting movement, muscle coordination, and posture. While there is no cure, various therapies can significantly improve a child's life by addressing specific challenges and promoting their overall development.

This section delves into three key therapies: Physical Therapy, Occupational Therapy, and Speech Therapy, exploring their goals and how they empower children with CP to reach their full potential.

Physical Therapy

Physical therapy forms the cornerstone of CP management. A physical therapist assesses a child's muscle tone, flexibility, balance, and movement patterns. They then design a personalized exercise program to improve motor skills. Through targeted exercises, therapists help children develop gross motor skills like walking, running, and jumping. For those with more severe limitations, therapists work on improving mobility and functional movements like transferring from sitting to standing.

- **Enhancing strength and coordination:** Strengthening exercises build muscle tone and improve coordination, allowing children with CP greater control over their movements. This not only improves their physical abilities but also boosts their confidence and independence.
- **Promoting balance and posture:** Balance and posture training are crucial for children with CP. Therapists use various techniques, including specific exercises and adaptive equipment, to help them maintain proper posture and improve their balance, reducing the risk of falls and injuries.

Occupational Therapy

Occupational Therapists (OTs) focus on helping children with CP develop the skills they need to perform daily living tasks independently. An OT assesses a child's needs and creates a therapy plan that is customized to individual needs of the patient.

- **Developing self-care skills:** This involves teaching children age-appropriate skills like dressing, bathing, grooming, and toileting. OTs also incorporate adaptive techniques and tools to make these tasks easier for children with limited mobility.
- **Improving fine motor skills:** OTs work on strengthening fine motor skills like grasping, manipulating objects, and writing. This can involve using specialized tools or adapting activities to allow children with CP to participate in creative play and academic pursuits.
- **Promoting independence:** The ultimate goal of occupational therapy is to empower children with CP to become as independent as possible in their daily lives. Therapists work on strategies and techniques that allow them to manage their routines and participate in activities they enjoy.

Speech Therapy

Speech therapy is crucial for children with CP who experience challenges with communication. A speech therapist evaluates a child's speech, language development, and swallowing abilities, and then designs a therapy plan that might address individual issues as needed.

- **Enhancing communication skills:** Therapists work on improving a child's ability to express themselves clearly, whether verbally or through alternative communication methods like sign language or assistive devices.

- **Promoting language development:** For children with speech delays, speech therapy focuses on building vocabulary, understanding language structure, and developing strong communication skills.
- **Addressing swallowing difficulties:** Some children with CP might experience swallowing problems. Speech therapists work on exercises and techniques to improve swallowing function and prevent complications.

By working collaboratively, these therapies create a holistic approach to managing CP. Physical therapy builds a strong foundation, occupational therapy empowers independence, and speech therapy gives children a voice. Through dedicated therapy and unwavering support, children with CP can overcome challenges, develop vital skills, and achieve their full potential.

The Therapeutic Team

Cerebral Palsy (CP) presents a unique set of challenges for children, affecting their movement, communication, and daily living skills. However, a well-coordinated therapeutic team can play a pivotal role in helping them reach their full potential.

This section explores the roles of different professionals involved in a child's therapy plan and emphasizes the importance of collaboration between therapists, educators, and parents to create a symphony of support.

The Essential Players

A child's therapeutic team for CP typically consists of several key professionals.

- **Physical Therapists:** These specialists evaluate a child's muscle tone, flexibility, balance, and movement patterns. They design individualized exercise programs to improve motor skills, strengthen muscles, and enhance coordination.
- **Occupational Therapists:** Occupational therapists (OTs) focus on promoting independence in daily living activities. They assess a child's needs and develop strategies for mastering self-care skills, improving fine motor skills like writing, and adapting activities to promote self-sufficiency.
- **Speech Therapists:** For children with CP who experience communication challenges, speech therapists are vital. They evaluate speech, language development, and swallowing abilities and design therapies to improve communication skills, promote language development, and address swallowing difficulties.
- **Rehabilitation Specialists:** This broader category can include specialists like developmental therapists, assistive technology specialists, and psychologists. They provide additional support in areas such as cognitive development, utilizing assistive devices, and managing emotional and social challenges associated with CP.

The Power of Collaboration

The magic happens when these professionals work together. Each therapist brings their unique expertise to the table, creating a comprehensive plan that addresses the child's physical, cognitive, and communication needs. Effective collaboration extends beyond the therapeutic team.

- **Therapists and Educators:** Communication and collaboration between therapists, teachers, and special education specialists ensure consistency in treatment approaches across school and home environments.
- **Therapists and Parents:** Parents are a child's first therapists and play a crucial role in implementing therapeutic strategies at home.

Therapists empower parents by providing training and resources to support their child's development.

- **Teamwork Makes the Dream Work:** When therapists, educators, and parents work together as a team, they create a unified approach that supports the child's holistic development and maximizes their chances of success.

Teamwork for Support

Imagine a child with CP struggling to communicate. The speech therapist equips them with communication tools, the occupational therapist helps them write, and the teacher incorporates these strategies into the classroom. This level of collaboration creates a symphony of support, where each note plays an essential role in creating a beautiful melody of progress for the child.

By fostering collaboration within the therapeutic team and including educators and parents, children with CP receive a holistic and coordinated approach to manage their condition. This collaborative spirit lays the foundation for a child's journey towards achieving their full potential and living a fulfilling life.

Comprehensive Therapy Plan

Cerebral Palsy (CP) presents a unique set of challenges for each child. Their needs may vary greatly, requiring a personalized therapy plan to maximize their potential.

This section explores the key steps involved in creating a comprehensive therapy plan – setting realistic goals, coordinating with other interventions, and monitoring progress – to build a bridge to success for your child.

Understanding Your Child's Needs

The first step is a thorough evaluation by a team of specialists, including doctors, therapists, and educators. This evaluation assesses your child's strengths, weaknesses, developmental level, and specific challenges related to CP. This information forms the foundation for crafting a personalized therapy plan.

Setting SMART Goals

Effective therapy plans involve setting **SMART** goals.

- **Specific:** Clearly define what you want to achieve. Instead of a vague goal like "improve communication," set a specific target like "increase the number of words used in expressive speech by x% within y months."
- **Measurable:** Track progress and quantify success. This allows you to adjust the plan as needed.
- **Attainable:** Set challenging yet achievable goals. Unrealistic goals can be discouraging for both you and your child.
- **Relevant:** Focus on goals that address your child's specific needs and align with their long-term aspirations.
- **Time-bound:** Set a timeframe for achieving each goal. This creates a sense of urgency and helps you measure progress.

Building a Cohesive Plan

Therapy needs to be integrated with other interventions your child might be receiving.

- **Complement Schoolwork:** Ensure therapy goals complement what your child is learning at school.

- **Incorporate Home Activities:** Therapists can suggest home activities and exercises that reinforce the therapy approaches used in sessions.
- **Coordinate with Other Specialists:** If your child receives additional therapies or interventions, ensure all specialists are aware of the overall plan and work together harmoniously.

Monitoring Progress and Making Adjustments

Monitoring progress is crucial for a successful therapy plan.

- **Regular Assessments:** Schedule regular evaluation sessions to track your child's progress toward goals.
- **Data Collection:** Document observations and track your child's advancement. This data can be vital when adjusting the plan.
- **Communicate with Therapists:** Open communication between parents and therapists is vital. Discuss any concerns you have and work together on refining the plan as needed.

A comprehensive therapy plan is a roadmap, not a rigid script. Flexibility is key to accommodate your child's changing needs and progress.

By setting SMART goals, coordinating with other interventions, and continuously monitoring progress, you can ensure your child's therapy plan acts as a bridge to success, empowering them to reach their full potential and live a fulfilling life.

17. THE JOURNEY THROUGH ADULTHOOD

Cerebral Palsy (CP) presents a unique set of challenges, but it does not define a person's potential. This section explores the possibilities and opportunities available for individuals with CP to live fulfilling and successful lives. By highlighting stories of successful adults with CP and fostering a spirit of hope and optimism, we can rewrite the narrative and empower those living with CP to embrace their potential.

Beyond the Diagnosis

CP encompasses a spectrum of severity, affecting each individual differently. While some individuals with CP may require significant assistance with daily activities, others may lead relatively independent lives. The key lies in focusing on possibilities, not limitations. Advancements in therapy, assistive technology, and social inclusion are creating a world where individuals with CP can thrive.

Success Stories Abound

Many individuals with CP have defied expectations and achieved remarkable things. Here are just a few examples:

- **Lauren Hill:** A renowned basketball player with CP, Lauren dominated college basketball before pursuing a successful career in motivational speaking and advocacy.
- **Jess Markt:** An Australian Paralympic gold medalist swimmer, Jess is a testament to the power of dedication and perseverance.
- **Stephen Hawking:** The world-renowned physicist, despite his severe limitations due to CP, made groundbreaking contributions to our understanding of the universe.

These stories showcase the diverse paths to success open to individuals with CP. They can pursue careers in academia, arts, sports, or any field that ignites their passion. Relationships, love, and independent living are all achievable with the right support systems in place.

Building a Supportive Environment

Creating a supportive environment is crucial for fostering hope and optimism. This includes:

- **Early Intervention:** Early diagnosis and access to therapy can significantly improve a child's outcomes.
- **Empowering Families:** Families play a pivotal role in advocating for their child's needs and fostering their independence.
- **Inclusive Communities:** Building inclusive communities that celebrate diversity and provide opportunities for individuals with CP is essential.

A Brighter Future

The future for individuals with CP is brimming with possibilities. Technological advancements promise new opportunities for communication, mobility, and independent living. A growing awareness of disability rights and inclusion is fostering a more accepting and supportive world.

Embracing Hope, Achieving Dreams

Living with CP may present challenges, but it does not have to limit one's potential. By focusing on strengths, celebrating achievements, and fostering a supportive environment, individuals with CP can rewrite the narrative. With unwavering hope and unwavering determination, they can achieve their dreams and live fulfilling lives, inspiring others along the way. The future is bright, and individuals with CP are ready to embrace it.

Resources

List of ten reputable websites in English focused on cerebral palsy from various countries:

United States: United Cerebral Palsy (UCP): A national organization providing information, resources, and advocacy for individuals with cerebral palsy. (Website: https://ucp.org/)

United Kingdom: Scope: A UK-based charity offering support, information, and advice for people with cerebral palsy and their families. (Website: https://www.scope.org.uk/)

Australia: Cerebral Palsy Alliance: A leading Australian organization providing services, support, and resources for people with cerebral palsy and their families. (Website: https://www.cpaustralia.com.au/)

Canada: Cerebral Palsy Canada: A national organization dedicated to supporting individuals with cerebral palsy through advocacy, research, and community programs. (Website: https://www.cerebralpalsy.ca/)

India: Trishla Foundation: A non-profit organization in India providing rehabilitation services, education, and support for children and adults with cerebral palsy. (Website: https://www.trishlafoundation.com/)

South Africa: Cerebral Palsy Association of South Africa (CPASA): A national organization offering support, information, and advocacy for individuals with cerebral palsy and their families. (Website: https://www.cerebralpalsysa.co.za/)

New Zealand: Cerebral Palsy Society of New Zealand: A charity organization dedicated to supporting and advocating for people with cerebral palsy and their families in New Zealand. (Website: https://www.cpsociety.org.nz/)

Ireland: Enable Ireland: A leading provider of services and support for children and adults with disabilities, including cerebral palsy, in Ireland. (Website: https://www.enableireland.ie/)

Singapore: Cerebral Palsy Alliance Singapore (CPAS): An organization offering early intervention, therapy, and support services for individuals with cerebral palsy and their families in Singapore. (Website: https://www.cpas.org.sg/)

Nigeria: Cerebral Palsy Foundation Nigeria: A non-governmental organization dedicated to providing education, therapy, and support for children with cerebral palsy and their families in Nigeria. (Website: https://www.cerebralpalsynigeria.org/)

ABOUT THE AUTHOR

Dr. A. Mitra is a retired medical doctor who has worked in the field of General Practice in Family Medicine in India and Australia for over 30 years. He completed his graduate education in India and then did further studies in Australia and UK. Currently he lives a private modest life and pursues his interests in reading and writing on various topics.

150